Computer Application in Pharmacy

Theory and Practical

for Second Semester Bachelor in Pharmacy

As per the latest syllabus prescribed by Pharmacy Council of India

W0235492

Computer Application in Pharmacy
Theory and Practical

for Second Semester Bachelor in Pharmacy

As per the latest syllabus prescribed by Pharmacy Council of India

Gaurav Agarwal M Pharma, PhD
Dean, Faculty of Pharmacy
RP Inderaprastha Institute of Technology
Karnal, Haryana

Parmeet Kaur M Tech (CSE)
Head, Department of CSE
RP Inderaprastha Institute of Technology
Karnal, Haryana

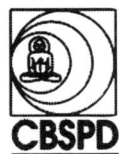

CBSPD

CBS Publishers & Distributors Pvt Ltd

New Delhi • Bengaluru • Chennai • Kochi • Kolkata • Lucknow • Mumbai
Hyderabad • Jharkhand • Nagpur • Patna • Pune • Uttarakhand

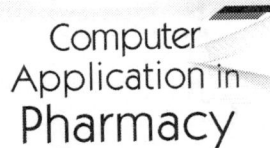

Computer
Application in
Pharmacy
Theory and Practical

ISBN: 978-81-948986-3-4

First Edition: 2021

Reprint: 2023, 2024, **2026**

Published by **Satish Kumar Jain** and produced by **Varun Jain** for

CBS Publishers & Distributors Pvt Ltd

4819/XI Prahlad Street, 24 Ansari Road, Daryaganj, New Delhi 110 002, India
Ph: 011-23289259, 23266838   Website: www.cbspd.com
                                e-mail: delhi@cbspd.com

Corporate Office: 204 FIE, Industrial Area, Patparganj, Delhi 110 092
Ph: 011-4934 4934   Fax: 011-4934 4935   e-mail: publishing@cbspd.com; publicity@cbspd.com

Branches

- **Bengaluru:** Seema House 2975, 17th Cross, K.R. Road, Banasankari 2nd Stage, Bengaluru 560 070, Karnataka, India
  Ph: +91-80-26771678/79   Fax: +91-80-26771680   e-mail: bangalore@cbspd.com

- **Chennai:** 18/8B, Subbarayan Street, Shenoy Nagar, Chennai 600 030, Tamil Nadu, India
  Ph: +91-44-42032115, 26681266   e-mail: chennai@cbspd.com

- **Kochi:** 42/1325, 1326, Power House Road, opposite KSEB, Power House, Ernakulam 682 018, Kochi, Kerala, India
  Ph: +91-484-4059061–65   Fax: +91-484-4059065   e-mail: kochi@cbspd.com

- **Kolkata:** 147, Hind Ceramics Compound, 1st Floor, Nilgunj Road, Belghoria, Kolkata-700 056, West Bengal, India
  Ph: +91-33-25633055–56   e-mail: kolkata@cbspd.com

- **Lucknow:** Basement, Khushnuma Complex, 7-Meerabai Marg (behind Jawahar Bhawan), Lucknow 226 001, UP, India
  Ph: +91-522-4000032   e-mail: tiwari.lucknow@cbspd.com

- **Mumbai:** PWD Shed. Gala No. 25/26, Ramchandra Bhatt Marg, Next to JJ Hospital Gate No. 2, Opp. Union Bank of India Noorbaug Mumbai-400 009, Maharashtra, India
  Ph: +91-22-66661880/89   e-mail: mumbai@cbspd.com

Representatives

- **Gujarat**   0-9879558667
- **Patna**   0-9334159340
- **Hyderabad** 0-9885175004
- **Pune**   0-9664372571
- **Jharkhand**   0-9811541605
- **Uttarakhand** 0-9716462459
- **Nagpur**   0-8692091830

Printed at Mudrak, Noida, UP, India

to

---

my loving parents
Mr Harbhajan Singh and Mrs Gurdev Kaur
my dear brother Lucky
and
my dear and loving husband Harjot Singh

— Parmeet Kaur

Preface

This book *Computer Application in Pharmacy* is designed specifically for B Pharmacy second semester students as per PCI (Pharmacy Council of India) course curriculum. This book covers wide areas and contains a comprehensive description of existing knowledge of computer applications. The book is a thoughtful compilation for beginners in pharmacy. The text not only deals with the basic concepts but also emphasizes technical and practical aspects of the subject. The book is primarily intended as textbook for students of pharmacy for degree and diploma courses. Being an interdisciplinary subject, it is today covering a wide range of interest, both among the students and the teaching communities. Taking this increasing interest into account, this book gives a comprehensives introduction to the subject.

The book contains numerous specimens, vivid illustrations, tables, diagrams and flow diagrams to present the ideas. The distinguishing feature is ample question bank at the end of the book. The structure and the content of the book have changed to reflect modern thinking and current university curricula throughout the world. The distinguishing feature is practical related to subject at the end of the book. In spite of great care, there might be some mistakes and deficiencies. We will be grateful for giving suggestions to improve. Please go through the content and send us mail at *gbitsian@rediffmail.com.*

Gaurav Agarwal

Parmeet Kaur

Acknowledgements

I am especially thankful to Shri RP Singal Ji, Chairman, RP Educational Trust, for his all time support and encouragement.

My special thanks to Er Bharat Singal, Secretary, RP Educational Trust, for inspiring us to bring out this book.

I am indebted to Dr Rajiv Singal, Vice Chairman, RP Educational Trust, and Shri DL Mittal, RPIIT Technical and Medical Campus, for their motivation.

I express my gratefulness to Mr YN Arjuna, Senior Vice President—Publishing, and Mr Satish K Jain, CMD, CBS Publishers and Distributors, for their sincere efforts.

I express my gratitude to my father Er VK Agarwal and my mother Asha Agarwal for their blessings and moral support.

Last but not least, I express my love to my wife Dr Shilpi and my loving kids Shreya and Vaidish for their all time inspiration and support. They are always a constant source of motivation in bringing out this achievement.

I thank my numerous students, whom I cannot possibly name individually, for their class interactions which have been the guiding spirit in selection of the subject matter and its logical arrangement.

Gaurav Agarwal

First of all I would like to thank God for giving me the strength to do work on this book.

Then, I would like to thank Dr Gaurav Agarwal, who helped me and guided me in the right way to do work and completion of book.

I would like to thank Er Bharat Singal, Secretary, RP Educational Trust, for inspiring us to bring out this book, and Shri DL Mittal, RPIIT Technical and Medical Campus, for his motivation.

In the end I would like to thank all my teachers and students.

Parmeet Kaur

Contents

Number System in Computers

COMPUTER

A computer is a programmable machine designed to perform sequence of operations to generate the desired output. It takes data as input, processes the data and produces the output. Earlier the computer was originally defined as a super fast calculator. It had the capacity to solve complex arithmetic and scientific problems at very high speed. But nowadays in addition to handling complex arithmetic computations, computers perform many other tasks like accepting, sorting, selecting, moving, comparing various types of information.

Computer is an advanced electronic device that takes raw data as input from the user and processes these data under the control of set of instructions (called program) and gives the result (output) and saves output for the future use. It can process both numerical and non-numerical (arithmetic and logical) calculations.

Functionality of a Computer

Any computer carries basic functions mentioned as

1. Takes data as input.
2. Stores the data or instructions in memory
3. Processes the data and generates the output.

Characteristics of a Computer

Some of the basic characteristics of computer are:

Speed: A computer is a very fast device. It can do calculations in just fractions of seconds. Computer can perform millions (1,000,000) of instructions and even more per second. Therefore, we determine the speed of computer in terms of microsecond or nanosecond.

Accuracy: The degree of accuracy of computer is very high and every calculation is performed with the same accuracy. Provided the input is correct, it performs the calculations with 100% accuracy.

Diligence: A computer is free from tiredness, lack of concentration, fatigue, etc. It can work for hours without creating any error. If millions of calculations are to be performed, a computer will perform every calculation with the same accuracy.

Versatility: A computer can perform different types of tasks and is a very versatile machine. A computer is very flexible in performing the jobs to be done.

Storage capability: The Computer has an in-built memory where it can store a large amount of data. It can store any type of data such as images, videos, text, audio, etc. Also it can store data in secondary storage devices.

No IQ: Computer is a dumb machine and it cannot do any work without instruction from the user. It performs the instructions at tremendous speed and with accuracy. It is you to decide what you want to do and in what sequence. So a computer cannot take its own decision as you can.

Computer Components

A computer can process data, pictures, sound and graphics. They can solve highly complicated problems quickly and accurately. A computer as shown in Figure performs basically five major computer operations or functions irrespective of their size and make (Fig. 1.1).

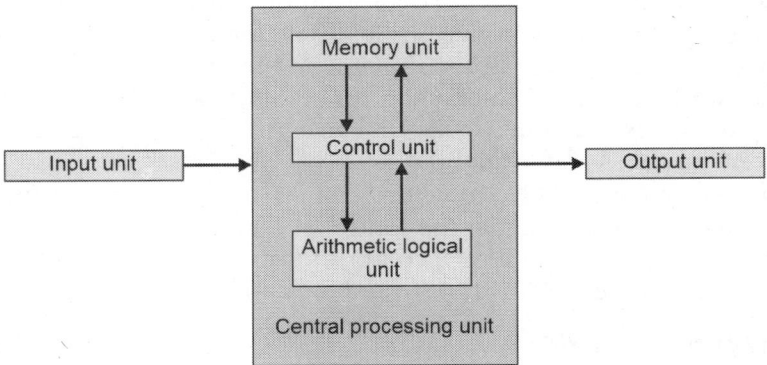

Fig. 1.1: Block diagram of computer

Input Unit

The input unit takes the data from the user and transfers the data to the central processing unit for processing. The input unit connects the external environment the computer system.

Central Processing Unit

The CPU also called the brain of computer which consists of following parts:

    a. Control unit: The control unit takes the responsibility of controlling all the operations of the entire computer system. The operations of input, processing and output are all done under the supervision of control unit.

    b. Arithmetic and logical unit: An arithmetic logic unit (ALU) is a combinational digital electronic circuit that performs arithmetic and bitwise operations on integer binary numbers. This is in contrast to a floating-point unit (FPU), which operates on floating point numbers. An ALU is a fundamental building block of many types of computing circuits, including the central processing unit (CPU) of computers, FPUs, and graphics processing units (GPUs). A single CPU, FPU or GPU may contain multiple ALUs.

NUMBER SYSTEM

A number system is the mathematical notation for representing numbers of a given set by using digits or other symbols in a consistent manner. A computer can understand the positional number system where there are only a few symbols called digits and these symbols represent different values depending on the position they occupy in the number. The value of any digit in a number can be determined by

i. The digit

ii. Its position in the number

iii. The base of the number system

A 'base' or a 'radix' is the number of different digits or combination of digits and letters that a system of counting uses to represent numbers.

The digit at the extreme left has the highest positional value and is generally called the Most Significant Digit, or in short MSD. Similarly, the digit occupying the extreme right position has the least positional value and is referred to as the Least Significant Digit or LSD.

Following are the different Number Systems

1. Decimal number system (Base 10)
2. Binary number system (Base 2)
3. Octal number system (Base 8)
4. Hexadecimal number system (Base 16)

Binary	Decimal	Octal	Hexadecimal
0000	00	0	0
0001	01	1	1
0010	02	2	2
0011	03	3	3
0100	04	4	4
0101	05	5	5
0110	06	6	6
0111	07	7	7
1000	08	10	8
1001	09	11	9
1010	10	12	A
1011	11	13	B
1100	12	14	C
1101	13	15	D
1110	14	16	E
1111	15	17	F

Decimal Number System

The decimal number system has ten digits 0 through 9. In decimal number system, the successive positions to the left of the decimal point represent units, tens, hundreds, thousands, and so on. The position of each digit in a decimal number indicates the magnitude of the quantity represented and can be assigned a weight. The weights for whole numbers are positive powers of ten that increases from right to left, beginning with $10^0 = 1$ that is $10^3\ 10^2\ 10^1\ 10^0$. For fractional numbers, the weights are negative powers of ten that decrease from left to right beginning with 10^{-1} that is $10^{-1}\ 10^{-2}\ 10^{-3}$. The value of a decimal number is the sum of digits after each digit has been multiplied by its weights as in following examples.

Express the decimal number 96 as a sum of the values of each digit.

The digit 9 has a weight of 10 which is 10 as indicated by its position. The digit 6 has a weight of 1 which is 10^0 as indicated by its position.

$$96 = (9 \times 10^1) + (6 \times 10^0)$$

Express the decimal number 625 as a sum of the values of each digit.

$$625 = (6 \times 10^2) + (2 \times 10^1) + (5 \times 10^0) = 600 + 20 + 5$$

Express the decimal number 625.25 as a sum of the values of each digit.

$$625.\,25 = (6 \times 10^2) + (2 \times 10^1) + (5 \times 10^0) + (2 \times 10^{-1}) + (5 \times 10^{-2}) = 600 + 20 + 5 + 0.2 + 0.05$$

Binary Number System

The **binary numbering system** is the most fundamental numbering system in all digital and computer based systems. It consists of two digits 0 and 1. Each digit position in a binary number represents a power of two. When we write a binary number, each binary digit is multiplied by an appropriate power of 2 which is based on their position in the number. The binary numbering system works on powers of two giving a binary to decimal conversion from base 2 to base 10.

In the binary numbering system, a binary number such as 1010101 is expressed with a string of '1's' and '0's' with each digit along the string from right to left having a value twice that of the previous digit.

Conversion between Decimal and Binary

Converting a number from binary to decimal is quite easy. All that is required is to find the decimal value of each binary digit position containing a 1 and add them up.

For example, convert $(10101)_2$ to its decimal equivalent as

$$10101_2 = [(1 \times 2^4) + (0 \times 2^3) + (1 \times 2^2) + (0 \times 2^1) + (1 \times 2^0)]_{10}$$
$$= (16 + 0 + 4 + 0 + 1)_{10}$$
$$= 21_{10}$$

Another example, convert $(11001)_2$ to its decimal equivalent as

$$11001_2 = [(1 \times 2^4) + (1 \times 2^3) + (0 \times 2^2) + (0 \times 2^1) + (1 \times 2^0)]_{10}$$
$$= (16 + 8 + 0 + 0 + 1)_{10}$$
$$= 25_{10}$$

The method for converting a decimal number to binary is one that can be used to convert from decimal to any number base. It involves using successive division by the radix until the dividend reaches 0. At each division, the remainder provides a digit of the converted number, starting with the least significant digit.

For example, convert 36_{10} to its binary equivalent as

$36/2 = 18$ remainder 0 (least significant digit)

$18/2 = 9$ remainder 0

$9/2 = 4$ remainder 1

$4/2 = 2$ remainder 0

$2/2 = 1$ remainder 0

$1/2 = 0$ remainder 1 (most significant digit)

The resulting binary number is 100100_2.

For example, convert 93_{10} to its binary equivalent as

$93/2 = 46$ remainder 1 (least significant digit)

$46/2 = 23$ remainder 0

$23/2 = 11$ remainder 1

$11/2 = 5$ remainder 1

$5/2 = 2$ remainder 1

$2/2 = 1$ remainder 0

$1/2 = 0$ remainder 1 (most significant digit)

The resulting binary number is 1011101_2.

Hexadecimal Number System

The hexadecimal number system has 16 digits and is used primarily as a compact way of displaying or writing binary numbers because it is very easy to convert between binary and hexadecimal. Hexadecimal is widely used in computer and microprocessor applications. The hexadecimal system has a base of sixteen it is composed of 16 digits and alphabetic characters. Each digit position represents a power of 16.

The reason for the common use of hexadecimal numbers is the relationship between the numbers 2 and 16. Sixteen is a power of 2 ($16 = 24$). Because of this relationship, four digits in a binary number can be represented with a single hexadecimal digit. This makes conversion between binary and hexadecimal numbers very easy, and hexadecimal can be used to write large binary numbers with much fewer digits.

The maximum 3-digits hexadecimal number is FFF or decimal 4095 and maximum 4-digit hexadecimal number is FFFF or decimal 65, 535.

When working with large digital systems, it is difficult to both read or write without producing errors especially when working with lots of 16 or 32 bit binary numbers. One common way of overcoming this problem is to arrange the binary numbers into groups or sets of four bits (4 bits). Four bits is called a nibble. A nibble is one hexadecimal digit, and is written using a symbol 0–9 or A-F. Two nibbles is a byte (8 bits). A nibble uses another type of numbering system also commonly used in computer and digital systems called **hexadecimal numbers**.

The main advantage of a **hexadecimal number** is that it is very compact and by using a base of 16 means that the number of digits used to represent a given number is usually less than in binary or decimal. Also, it is quick and easy to convert between hexadecimal numbers and binary.

Conversion

1. Binary to hexadecimal

Grouping method is used to change a number from binary to hexadecimal. Separate a binary number into groups of four digits starting from the right. Groups are then converted to hexadecimal digits from 0 to F. To change from hexadecimal, the reverse is done. Grouping is usually removed after converting hexadecimal digits to binary (Table 1.1).

Table 1.1: Conversion of binary to hexadecimal

Binary	Groupings				Hexadecimal
01100101			0110	0101	65
010010110110		0100	1011	0110	4B6
1101011101011010	1101	0111	0101	1010	D75A

2. Hexadecimal to decimal

One way to find the decimal equivalent of a hexadecimal number is to first convert the hexadecimal number to binary and then convert from binary to decimal.

Convert the hexadecimal number 1C to decimal:

1 C

$0001\ 1100 = 2^4 + 2^3 + 2^2 = 16 + 8 + 4 = 28$

3. Decimal to hexadecimal

Repeated division of a decimal number by 16 will produce the equivalent hexadecimal number, formed by the remainders of the divisions. The first remainder produced is the least significant digit (LSD). Each successive division by 16 yields a remainder that becomes a digit in the equivalent hexadecimal number. When a quotient has a fractional part, the fractional part is multiplied by the divisor to get the remainder.

Convert the decimal number 650 to hexadecimal by repeated division by 16:

$650/16 = 40.625$ $0.625 \times 16 = 10 = A$ (LSD)

$40/16 = 2.5$ $0.5 \times 16 = 8 = 8$

$2/16 = 0.125$ $0.125 \times 16 = 2 = 2$ (MSD)

The hexadecimal number is 28A

*And another method to solve **decimal to hexadecimal** is given below:*

16	650	
16	40	10
16	2	8
	0	2

Hence the hexadecimal number is 2 8 10, i.e. 28A (because 10 = A in hexadecimal).

OCTAL NUMBERS

The octal number system is the base 8 number system and uses the digits 0 to 7. Like the hexadecimal system, the octal system provides a convenient way to express binary numbers and codes. However, it is used less frequently than hexadecimal in conjunction with computers and microprocessors to express binary quantities for input and output purposes.

To count above 7, begin another column and start over: 10, 11, 12, 13, 14, 15, 16, 17, 20, 21 and so on. Counting in octal is similar to counting in decimal, except that the digits 8 and 9 are not used.

The **octal numbering system** is very similar in principle to the previous hexadecimal numbering system except that in octal, a binary number is divided up into groups of only 3 bits, with each group or set of bits having a distinct value of between 000 (0) and 111 ($4 + 2 + 1 = 7$). Octal numbers therefore have a range of just '8' digits, (0, 1, 2, 3, 4, 5, 6, 7) making them a Base 8 numbering system and therefore, q is equal to '8'.

Then the main characteristics of an **octal numbering system** is that there are only 8 distinct counting digits from 0 to 7 with each digit having a weight or value of just 8 starting from the least significant bit (LSB). In the earlier days of computing, octal numbers and the octal numbering system was very popular for counting inputs and outputs because as it works in counts of eight, inputs and outputs were in counts of eight, a byte at a time.

As the base of an **octal numbers** system is 8 (base 8), which also represents the number of individual numbers used in the system, the subscript 8 is used to identify a number expressed in octal (Table 1.2).

Octal Numbers

Convert octal number 2574 in decimal number.

Weight $\qquad 8^3 \ 8^2 \ 8^1 \ 8^0$

Octal number $\qquad 2\ 5\ 7\ 4$

2574

$(2 \times 8^3) + (5 \times 8^2) + (7 \times 8^1) + (4 \times 8^0) = 1404$

Table 1.2: Octal numbers

Decimal number	3 Bit binary number	Octal number
0	000	0
1	001	1
2	010	2
3	011	3
4	100	4
5	101	5
6	110	6
7	111	7
8	001 000	10 (1 + 0)
9	001 001	11 (1 + 1)

Continuing upwards in groups of three

Conversion

1. Decimal to octal

It is a method of converting a decimal number to an octal number is the repeated division by 8 method, which is similar to the method. It is used to convert decimal numbers to binary or to hexadecimal.

Convert the decimal number 359 to octal. Each successive division by 8 yields a remainder that becomes a digit in the equivalent octal number. The first remainder generated is the least significant digit (LSD).

$359/8 = 44.875$ $0.875 \times 8 = 7$ (LSD)

$44/8 = 5.5$ $0.5 \times 8 = 4$

$5/8 = 0.625$ $0.625 \times 8 = 5$ (MSD)

The number is 547

2. Octal to binary

It is very easy to convert octal to binary because each digit can be represented by a 3 bit binary number.

Octal –>Binary conversion

Octal digit	0	1	2	3	4	5	6	7
Binary	000	001	010	011	100	101	110	111

Convert the octal numbers 23, i.e. 23 and 570 will come:

Octal digit	2	3	5	7	0
Binary	**010**	**011**	**101**	**111**	**000**

A FEW MORE EXAMPLE OCTAL TO BINARY

a. 1573_8

Solution:

1573_8

$= 001\ 101\ 111\ 011$

$= 1101111011_2$

Hence the required binary number is 1101111011.

b. 64.175_8

Solution:

64.175_8

$= 110\ 100\ .\ 001\ 111\ 101$

$= 110100.001111101_2$

Hence the required binary number is 110100.001111101.

3. Binary to octal conversion

It is the reverse of the octal to binary conversion.

Convert the following binary numbers to octal:

110		111	011	110	100
6		7	3	6	4

= 67364

A FEW MORE EXAMPLE BINARY TO OCTAL

a. 1110101110_2

Solution:

001110101110

= 001 110 101 110

= 1656_8

Hence the required octal equivalent is 1656.

b. 111101.01101_2

Solution:

111101.011010₂

= 75.32_8

Hence the required octal equivalent is 75.32.

Binary Addition and Subtraction

The addition and subtraction of the binary number system are similar to that of the decimal number system. The only difference is that the decimal number system consists the digit from 0–9 and their base is 10 whereas the binary number system consists only two digits (0 and 1) which make their operation easier. The addition and subtraction of binary number systems are explained below in details.

Binary Addition

The binary number system uses only two digits 0 and 1 due to which their addition is simple. There are four basic operations for binary addition, as mentioned above (Table 1.3).

Table 1.3: Binary addition

Case	A + B	Sum	Carry
1	0 + 0	0	0
2	0 + 1	1	0
3	1 + 0	1	0
4	1 + 1	0	1

In fourth case, a binary addition is creating a sum of (1 + 1 = 10), i.e. 0 is written in the given column and a carry of 1 over to the next column.

EXAMPLE ADDITION

i. 10101 and 11011

Solution:

10101 and 11011
1 1 1 1   Carry overs
1 0 1 0 1
<u>1 1 0 1 1</u>
1 1 0 0 0 0

ii. 11001 and 111

Solution:

11001 and 111
1 1 1 1   Carry overs
1 1 0 0 1
<u>   1 1 1</u>
1 0 0 0 0 0

iii. 10101.101 and 1101.011

Solution:
10101.101 and 1101.011

   1 1 1 1 1 1   Carry overs
1 0 1 0 1 . 1 0 1
<u> 1 1 0 1 . 0 1 1</u>
1 0 0 0 1 1 . 0 0 0

iv. 111.0111 and 10011.001

Solution:

111.0111 and 10011.001
   1 1 1 1 1   Carry overs
   1 1 1 . 0 1 1 1
<u>1 0 0 1 1 . 0 0 1</u>
1 1 0 1 0 . 1 0 0 1

Note: Carefully that 10 + 1 = 11, which is equivalent to 2 + 1 = 3 (the next binary number after 10).

Binary Subtraction

The subtraction of the binary digit depends on the four basic operations (Table 1.4).

Case	A + B	Sum	Carry
Table 1.4: Binary subtraction			
1	0 − 0	0	0
2	1 − 0	1	0
3	1 − 1	0	0
4	0 − 1	0	1

The above first three operations are easy to understand as they are identical to decimal subtraction. The fourth operation can be understood with the logic two minus one is one.

EXAMPLE SUBTRACTION

i. 101 from 1001

Solution:

101 from 1001

   1 Borrow

  1 0 0 1

    1 0 1

   1 0 0

ii. 111 from 1000

Solution:

111 from 1000

   1 Borrow

1 0 0 0

  1 1 1

0 0 0 1

iii. 1010101.10 from 1111011.11

Solution:

1010101.10 from 1111011.11

       1 Borrow

1 1 1 1 0 1 1 . 1 1

1 0 1 0 1 0 1 . 1 0

 1 0 0 1 1 0 . 0 1

iv. 11010.101 from 101100.011

Solution:

11010.101 from 101100.011

1   1   1   Borrow

1 0 1 1 0 0 . 0 1 1

 1 1 0 1 0 . 1 0 1

 1 0 0 0 1 . 1 1 0

$0011010 - 001100 = 00001110$

$$
\begin{array}{r}
1\ 1 \quad\quad \text{borrow}\\
0\ 0\ \cancel{1}\ \cancel{1}\ 0\ 1\ 0 = 26_{10}\\
-\ 0\ 0\ 0\ 1\ 1\ 0\ 0 = 12_{10}\\
\hline
0\ 0\ 0\ 1\ 1\ 1\ 0 = 14_{10}
\end{array}
$$

1's Complement Binary Number

The **ones' complement** of a binary number is defined as the value obtained by inverting all the bits in the binary representation of the number (swapping 0s for 1s and *vice versa*). The ones' complement of the number then behaves like the negative of the original number in some arithmetic operations. To within a constant (of "1), the ones' complement behaves like the negative of the original number with binary addition. However, unlike 2's complement, these numbers have not seen widespread use because of issues such as the offset of "1, that negating zero results in a distinct negative zero bit pattern, less simplicity with arithmetic borrowing, etc. (Table 1.5).

Table 1.5: 1's complement binary number				
Given number				
1	0	1	0	1
0	1	0	1	1
1's complement				

2's Complement

The 2's complement of binary number is obtained by adding 1 to the least significant bit (LSB) of 1's complement of the number (Table 1.6).

2's complement = 1's complement + 1

Example of 2's complement is as follows.

Table 1.6: 2's complement binary number				
Given number				
1	0	1	0	1
0	1	0	1	0
1's complement				
Add 1 +				1
0	1	0	1	1

In Binary Addition Using 1's Complement

We discuss the following cases under this.

Case I: When the positive number has greater magnitude.

In this case addition of numbers is performed after taking 1's complement of the negative number and the end-around carry of the sum is added to the least significant bit.

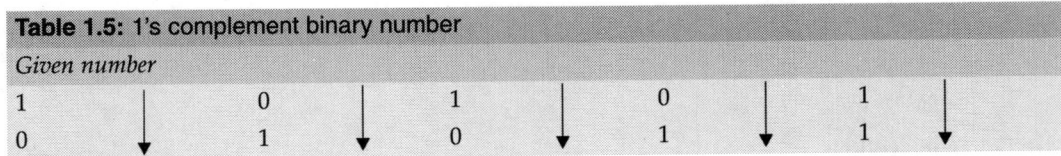

EXAMPLE FIND THE SUM OF THE FOLLOWING BINARY NUMBERS

   i. **+1110 and −1101**
   Solution:
   +1110   ⇒   0̲1110

$-1101 \Rightarrow \underline{1}0010$ (taking 1's complement)

$\underline{0}0000$

1 carry

$\underline{0}0001$

Hence the required sum is + 0001.

ii. +1101 and −1011

(Assume that the representation is in a signed 5-bit register).

Solution:

$+1101 \Rightarrow \underline{0}1101$

$-1011 \Rightarrow \underline{1}0100$ (taking 1's complement)

$\underline{0}0001$

1 carry

$\underline{0}0010$

Hence the required sum is + 0010.

Case II: When the negative number has greater magnitude.

In this case the addition is carried in the same way as in case 1 but there will be non end-around carry. The sum is obtained by taking 1's complement of the magnitude bits of the result and it will be negative.

The following examples will illustrate this method in binary addition using 1's complement

Find the sum of the following binary numbers represented in a sign-plus-magnitude 5-bit register:

i. +1010 and −1100

Solution:

$+1010 \Rightarrow \underline{0}1010$

$-1100 \Rightarrow \underline{1}0011$ (1's complement)

$\underline{1}1101$

Hence the required sum is − 0010.

Binary Addition using 2's Complement

When negative numbers are expressed in binary addition using 2's complement the addition of binary numbers becomes easier. This operation is almost similar to that in 1's complement system and is explained with examples given below:

We consider the following cases.

Case I: When the positive number has a greater magnitude.

In this case the carry which will be generated is discarded and the final result is the result of addition.

In a 5-bit register find the sum of the following by using 2's complement

i. –1011 and –0101

Solution:

+1 0 1 1   ⇒   0 1 0 1 1

–0 1 0 1   ⇒   1 1 0 1 1   (2's complement)

(Carry 1 discarded)   0 0 1 1 0

Hence the sum is + 0110.

ii. +0111 and –0011.

Solution:

+0 1 1 1   ⇒   0 0 1 1 1

–0 0 1 1   ⇒   1 1 1 0 1

(Carry 1 discarded)   0 0 1 0 0

Hence the sum is + 0100.

Case II: When the negative number is greater.

When the negative numbers is greater no carry will be generated in the sign bit. The result of addition will be negative and the final result is obtained by taking 2's complement of the magnitude bits of the result.

In a 5-bit register find the sum of the following by using 2's complement

i. +0 0 1 1 and –0 1 0 1

Solution:

+0 0 1 1   ⇒   0 0 0 1 1

–0 1 0 1   ⇒   1 1 0 1 1   (2's complement)

                       1 1 1 1 0

2's complement of 1110 is (0001 + 0001) or 0010.

Hence the required sum is –0010.

ii. +0 1 0 0 and –0 1 1 1

Solution:

+0 1 0 0   ⇒   0 0 1 0 0

–0 1 1 1   ⇒   1 1 0 0 1   (2's complement)

                       1 1 1 0 1

2's complement of 1101 is 0011.

Hence the required sum is –0011.

Subtraction by 1's Complement

The steps to be followed in subtraction by 1's complement are:

i. To write down 1's complement of the subtrahend.

ii. To add this with the minuend.

iii. If the result of addition has a carry-over then it is dropped and an 1 is added in the last bit.

iv. If there is no carry-over, then 1's complement of the result of addition is obtained to get the final result and it is negative.

Evaluate

i. 110101–100101

1's complement of 10011 is 011010. Hence

Minuend		1 1 0 1 0 1
1's complement of subtrahend		0 1 1 0 1 0
Carry-over	1	0 0 1 1 1 1
		1
		0 1 0 0 0 0

The required difference is 10000

ii. 101011–111001

Solution:

1's complement of 111001 is 000110. Hence

Minuend	1 0 1 0 1 1
1's complement	0 0 0 1 1 0
	1 1 0 0 0 1

Hence the difference is –1 1 1 0

iii. 1011.001–110.10

Solution:

1's complement of 0110.100 is 1001.011 Hence

Minuend		1 0 1 1 . 0 0 1
1's complement of subtrahend		1 0 0 1 . 0 1 1
Carry-over	1	0 1 0 0 . 1 0 0
		1
		0 1 0 0 . 1 0 1

Hence the required difference is 100.101

iv. 10110.01–11010.10

Solution

1's complement of 11010.10 is 00101.01

1 0 1 1 0 . 0 1
0 0 1 0 1 . 0 1
1 1 0 1 1 . 1 0

Hence the required difference is –00100.01, i.e. –100.01

Subtraction by 2's Complement

With the help of subtraction by 2's complement method we can easily subtract two binary numbers.

The operation is carried out by means of the following steps:

i. At first, 2's complement of the subtrahend is found.
ii. Then it is added to the minuend.
iii. If the final carry-over of the sum is 1, it is dropped and the result is positive.
iv. If there is no carry-over, the two's complement of the sum will be the result and it is negative.

Evaluate

i. 110110–10110

Solution:

The numbers of bits in the subtrahend is 5 while that of minuend is 6. We make the number of bits in the subtrahend equal to that of minuend by taking a '0' in the sixth place of the subtrahend.

Now, 2's complement of 010110 is (101101 + 1), i.e.101010. Adding this with the minuend.

$$
\begin{array}{ll}
1\ 10110 & \text{Minuend} \\
\underline{1\ 01010} & \text{2's complement of subtrahend} \\
\text{Carry-over 1} \quad 1\ 00000 & \text{Result of addition}
\end{array}
$$

After dropping the carry-over we get the result of subtraction to be 100000.

ii. 10110–11010

Solution:

2's complement of 11010 is (00101 + 1) i.e. 00110. Hence

$$
\begin{array}{ll}
\text{Minuend} & 10110 \\
\text{2's complement of subtrahend} & \underline{00110} \\
\text{Result of addition} & 11100
\end{array}
$$

As there is no carry-over, the result of subtraction is negative and is obtained by writing the 2's complement of 11100, i.e. (00011 + 1) or 00100.

Hence the difference is – 100.

iii. 1010.11–1001.01

Solution:

2's complement of 1001.01 is 0110.11. Hence

$$
\begin{array}{ll}
\text{Minuend} & 1010.11 \\
\text{2's complement of subtrahend} & \underline{0110.11} \\
\text{Carry-over} & 1\ 0001.10
\end{array}
$$

After dropping the carry-over we get the result of subtraction as 1.10.

iv. 10100.01–11011.10

Solution:

2's complement of 11011.10 is 00100.10. Hence

$$
\begin{array}{ll}
\text{Minuend} & 10100.01 \\
\text{2's complement of subtrahend} & \underline{01100.10} \\
\text{Result of addition} & 11000.11
\end{array}
$$

As there is no carry-over the result of subtraction is negative and is obtained by writing the 2's complement of 11000.11.

Hence the required result is – 00111.01.

Binary Multiplication

It is similar as multiplication of decimal numbers. The binary multiplication is much easier as it contains only 0s and 1s. The four fundamental rules for binary multiplication are

$0 \times 0 = 0$

$0 \times 1 = 0$

$1 \times 0 = 0$

$1 \times 1 = 1$

The multiplication of two binary numbers can be performed by using two common methods, namely partial product addition and shifting, and using parallel multipliers.

Note that since binary operates in base 2, the multiplication rules we need to remember are those that involve 0 and 1 only.

Unsigned binary numbers multiplication process

EXAMPLES FOR BINARY MULTIPLICATION

i. 10111 by 1101

Solution:

```
        10111
         1101
        10111      ← First partial product
        10111
      1110011      ← First intermediate sum
        10111
    100101011      ← Final sum.
```

Hence the required product is 100101011.

ii. 11011.101 by 101.111

```
      11011.101
        101.111
      11011.101
     110111.01      ← First partial product
    1010010 111     ← First intermediate sum
     1101110 1
    11000001 011    ← Second intermediate sum
    11011101
   110011110 011    ← Third intermediate sum
```

$$\underline{\quad 1101111}$$
$$10100010010 \ 011$$

Hence the required result is 10100010.010011.

From the above multiplication, partial products are generated for each digit in the multiplier. Then all these partial products are added to produce the final product value. In the partial product multiplication, when the multiplier bit zero, the partial product is zero, and when the multiplier bit is 1, the resulted partial product is the multiplicand.

As similar to the decimal numbers, each successive partial product is shifted one position left relative to the preceding partial product before summing all partial products.

Therefore, this multiplication uses n-shifts and adds to multiply n-bit binary number. The combinational circuit implemented to perform such multiplication is called an array multiplier or combinational multiplier.

Binary Division

To perform a binary number division, we need to follow the same process as we do for dividing regular numbers, but in this case, we only need to decide if it is going to be a 1 or a 0.

To divide two numbers which result is an exact division, we basically need to follow four steps: division, multiplication, subtraction, and next digit.

Letus say that we want to divide 18 by 3, which in binary will be 10010 divided by 00011 (or 11, it is the same).

$$11\sqrt{10010}$$

First, we need to identify digit by digit. Is 11 less or equal than 1? No, so we get another digit. Is 11 less or equal than 10? No, so we repeat and get another digit. Is 11 less or equal than 100? Yes, so in this case we do not need to think how many times can 100 be divided by 11, instead, we just add a 1 to the product.

$$1$$
$$11\sqrt{10010}$$

100 can be divided by 11

Now we need to multiply 11 by the product 1. Then, we need to subtract 11 from the digits we have considered so far, which in this case are three, 100:

$$1$$
$$11\sqrt{10010}$$
$$\underline{\quad 11}$$

Multiply 11 by the product 1 to get 11
Remember that 0 minus 1 requires us to carry a 1 from the next digit.

$$1$$
$$11\sqrt{10010}$$
$$\underline{\quad 11}$$

Carry a 1 to the next digit

In this particular case, we can carry enough 1's to complete the subtraction, so we need to consider the subtraction as a whole:

```
        1
11√10010
    11
```

Few more examples of binary division:

i. 11001 ÷ 101

Solution:

```
101)  11001  (101
      101
       101
       101
```

Hence the quotient is 101

ii. 11101.01 ÷ 1100

Solution:

```
1100)  11101.01  (10.0111
       1100
        10101
        1100
         0010
         1100
          1100
          1100
```

Hence the quotient is 10.0111

iii. 10110.1 ÷ 1101

Solution:

```
1101)  10110.1  (1.101
       1101
        10011
        1101
         11000
         1101
          1011
```

Thus, the quotient is 1.101 up to 3 places of binary point and the remainder is 1.011.

iv. 101.11 ÷ 111

Solution:

```
111) 101.11  (0.11
      11 1
      10 01
       1 11
         10
```

Thus, the quotient is 0.11 up to 2 places of binary point and the remainder is 0.1.

ISOLATED KEY POINTS

- **Natural numbers:** The numbers 1, 2, 3, 4.... are called natural numbers or positive integers.
- **Whole numbers:** The numbers 0, 1, 2, 3.... are called whole numbers. Whole numbers include "0".
- **Integers:** The numbers .... –3, –2, –1, 0, 1, 2, 3,.... are called integers. You will see questions on integers in almost all the exams where you see number system aptitude questions.
- **Negative integers:** The numbers –1, –2, –3, ... are called negative integers.
- **Positive fractions:** The numbers (2/3), (4/5), (7/8) ... are called positive fractions.
- **Negative fractions:** The numbers –(6/8), –(7/19), –(12/17) ... are called negative fractions.
- **Rational numbers:** Any number which is a positive or negative integer or fraction, or zero is called a rational number. A rational number is one which can be expressed in the following format ⇒(a/b) , where b ≠ 0 and a and b are positive or negative integers.
- **Irrational numbers:** An infinite non-recurring decimal number is known as an irrational number. These numbers cannot be expressed in the form of a proper fraction a/b where b ≠ 0, e.g. $\sqrt{2}$, Π, etc.
- **Surds:** Any root of a number, which cannot be exactly found is called a surd. Essentially, all surds are irrational numbers, e.g. $\sqrt{2}$, $\sqrt{5}$, etc.
- **Even numbers:** The integers which are divisible by 2 are called even numbers, e.g. –4, 0, 2, 16, etc.
- **Odd numbers:** The integers which are not divisible by 2 are odd numbers e.g. –7, –15, 5, 9, etc.
- **Prime numbers:** Those numbers, which are divisible only by themselves and 1, are called prime numbers. In other words, a number, which has only two factors, 1 and itself, is called a prime number, e.g. 2, 3, 5, 7, etc.

PRACTICE QUESTIONS

Long Answer Type Questions

1. What is computer? Explain the characteristics of computer.

2. Explain the block diagram of computer.

3. Explain number system.

4. Explain the conversion of binary too hexadecimal.

5. What are the components of computer? Explain with block diagram.

6. Comparison between binary, decimal and hexadecimal numbers.

7. Define 2's complement with example?

OBJECTIVE TYPE QUESTIONS

1. Which of the following numbers is divisible by 2?
   a. 178653   b. 164857
   c. 176485   d. 178560

2. Simplify the expression using BODMAS rule: (3/2) of (4/7) {(10 × 3) – (8 × 2)}
   a. 6   b. 12
   c. 18   d. 14

3. The product of 40 odd numbers is:
   a. Even   b. Odd
   c. 625   d. Can't say

4. The six digit number 54321A is divisible by 9 where A is a single digit whole number. Find A.
   a. 0   b. 2
   c. 4   d. 3

5. The seven digit number 43567X is divisible by 3, where X is a single digit whole number. Find X.
   a. 2   b. 5
   c. 8   d. All of these

6. Find the greatest three number which is multiple of 7.
   a. 993   b. 995
   c. 994   d. None of these

7. Find the greatest 6-digit number, which is a multiple of 12.
   a. 999980   b. 999990
   c. 999984   d. None of these

8. Find the smallest three number which is a multiple of 7.
   a. 103   b. 105
   c. 98   d. None of these

9. Simplify the expression using BODMAS rule (3/7) of (4/5) of 20 (252–242)
   a. 336   b. 168
   c. 84   d. None of these

10. **Simplify the expression using BODMAS rule $(105 + 206) - 550 \div 52 + 10$**

    a. 399   b. 289

    c. 298   d. 299

ANSWERS KEY

1. Option d

A number is divisible by 2 if the last digit of the number is 0 or a multiple of 2. Therefore only 178560 is divisible by 2. So, answer is option d.

2. Option b

Applying BODMAS rule $= (3/2)$ of $(4/7)$ {30–16} $= (12/14) \times 14 = 12$ Therefore, the correct answer is option b.

3. Option b

The product of 40 odd numbers will give an odd number. So answer is option b.

4. Option d

A number is divisible by 9, when the sum of its digits is divisible by 9. Here, $5 + 4 + 3 + 2 + 1 + A = 15 + A$ should be divisible by 9. Therefore, $A = 3$ gives $15 + 3 = 18$ as the sum of digits, which is divisible by 9. So, answer is option d.

5. Option d

A number is divisible by 3 when sum of its digits is divisible by 3. Here, sum of digits $= 4 + 3 + 5 + 6 + 7 + X = 25 + X$. So, X can be 2, 5, 8 which gives the sum 27, 30 and 33 respectively. Therefore, X has 3 values here, for which the number is divisible by 3. So, the answer is option d.

6. Option c

Greatest three digits number $= 999$. When 999 is divided by 7, the remainder will be 5. Required number $= 999 - 5 = 994$.

7. Option d

Greatest six-digit number is 999999. Divide this number by 12 and get remainder as 3. Since the remainder is 3, if you subtract 3 from the number, the remaining number will be a multiple of 12. So the greatest such number will be $999999 - 3 = 999996$

8. Option b

Smallest three digit number $=100$. Divide this number by 7 and get the remainder as 2. If you subtract 2 from the number the remaining number will be a multiple of 7, $100 - 2 = 98$ which is two digit number. Now if we add 7 so that we get the smallest three digit number which is a multiple of 7. Required number $= 98 + 7 = 105$

9. Option a

$(3/7) \times (4/5)$ of 20 (625–576) $\Rightarrow (3/7) \times (4/5) \times 20 \times 49 = 336$

10. Option d

$(105 + 206) - 550 \div 52 + 10$

$= 311 - 550 \div 25 + 10$

$= 311 - 22 + 10$

Number System in Computers in Place of Concept of Information System and Software

INFORMATION GATHERING

Information gathering is the act of collecting information from various sources through various means. It is an advanced skill which requires the training and education of personnel in the procedures and methods of gathering information from sources that are of higher level than ordinary sources.

In general practice, information gathering is the collection of data for dealing with the individual's or the organization's current situation. More data means more and better ways of dealing with the current situation.

Information gathering is an assignment of the research specialist within the organization's intelligence department. They are the personnel properly trained and equipped to carry out the research tasks in the most efficient manner.

In order to implement a good information gathering design, a step-by-step approach is advisable for any researcher to follow:

1. **Analyzing the problem:** The researcher needs to identify the purpose and the process of the research he is doing. For who is he doing it and why? These questions and more needs to be answered right at the start of the research.

2. **Identifying the sections of the information gathering:** Before going through with the process of information gathering, a sectioning of the general outline of the task can be helpful. Sections such as those classifying the recipients of the data, the detailing of the specific questions that needs to be answered, and also the setting of the knowledge levels of the team members involved facilitates an easier to follow research program.

3. **After the outline of the research task:** The researcher may then set the actual plan of activities needed to carry out the information gathering tasks. Questions such as: Where to go to for the research? What materials need to be invested in? What skills are needed to be implemented? And the details of the research materials like the availability, languages, location and accessibility needs some suasion.

4. **The gathering methods and tools:** The tools that are involved in information gathering such as data storage devices and publications have their own set of required skills that the researcher must readily possess or is capable of having. Languages contained in publications could pose a problem and data storage devices could have proprietary names. And names, as we all know in the computer industry means lots of adjustments.

5. **Begin the gathering:** During the gathering of the data, the researcher encounters various amounts of information that may or may not be relevant to the present subject of the research. He must sift through all of these carefully.
6. **Review and record the data obtained:** A recording that includes everything from the start to the end of the gathering process must be set in writing to provide all the information that the organization needs.
7. The information gathering strategy consists of identifying information sources, evolving a method of obtaining information from the identified sources and using an information flow model of organization. The main sources of information are users of the system, forms and documents used in the organization, procedure manuals, rule books, etc. reports used by the organization.

Requirement and Feasibility Analysis

Feasibility analysis answers two main questions:
   1. Can this approach to the solution work?
   2. Is the approach worthwhile, that is, do its benefits exceed its costs?

Requirements are the basis for answering both these questions. Satisfying the requirements provides measurable value (or benefits) by solving a problem, taking an opportunity, or meeting a challenge. A solution provides value if and only if it satisfies the requirements.

The feasibility study is basically the test of the proposed system in the light of its workability, meeting user's requirements, effective use of resources and of course, the cost effectiveness. These are categorized as technical, operational, economic and schedule feasibility. The main goal of feasibility study is not to solve the problem but to achieve the scope. In the process of feasibility study, the cost and benefits are estimated with greater accuracy to find the return on investment (ROI). This also defines the resources needed to complete the detailed investigation. The result is a feasibility report submitted to the management. This may be accepted or accepted with modifications or rejected. The system cycle proceeds only if the management accepts it.

Detailed System Study

The detailed investigation of the system is carried out in accordance with the objectives of the proposed system. This involves detailed study of various operations performed by a system and their relationships within and outside the system. During this process, data are collected on the available files, decision points and transactions handled by the present system. Interviews, on-site observation and questionnaire are the tools used for detailed system study. Using the following steps it becomes easy to draw the exact boundary of the new system under consideration:

   i. Keeping in view the problems and new requirements
   ii. Workout the pros and cons including new areas of the system.

All the data and the findings must be documented in the form of detailed data flow diagrams (DFDs), data dictionary, logical data structures and miniature specification. The main points to be discussed in this stage are:

Specification of what the new system is to accomplish based on the user requirements.

i. Functional hierarchy showing the functions to be performed by the new system and their relationship with each other.

ii. Functional network, which are similar to function hierarchy but they highlight the functions which are common to more than one procedure.

iii. List of attributes of the entities—these are the data items which need to be held about each entity (record).

System Analysis

Systems analysis is a process of collecting factual data, understand the processes involved, identifying problems and recommending feasible suggestions for improving the system functioning. This involves studying the business processes, gathering operational data, understand the information flow, finding out bottlenecks and evolving solutions for overcoming the weaknesses of the system so as to achieve the organizational goals. System analysis also includes subdividing of complex process involving the entire system, identification of data store and manual processes.

The major objectives of systems analysis are to find answers for each business process: What is being done, how is it being done, who is doing it, when is he doing it, why is it being done and how can it be improved? It is more of a thinking process and involves the creative skills of the system analyst. It attempts to give birth to a new efficient system that satisfies the current needs of the user and has scope for future growth within the organizational constraints. The result of this process is a logical system design. Systems analysis is an iterative process that continues until a preferred and acceptable solution emerges.

System Design

Based on the user requirements and the detailed analysis of the existing system, the new system must be designed. This is the phase of system designing. It is the most crucial phase in the developments of a system. The logical system design arrived at as a result of systems analysis is converted into physical system design. Normally, the design proceeds in two stages:

i. Preliminary or general design
ii. Structured or detailed design

Preliminary or general design: In the preliminary or general design, the features of the new system are specified. The costs of implementing these features and the benefits to be derived are estimated. If the project is still considered to be feasible, we move to the detailed design stage.

Structured or detailed design: In the detailed design stage, computer oriented work begins in earnest. At this stage, the design of the system becomes more structured. Structure design is a blue print of a computer system solution to a given problem having the same components and interrelationships among the same components as the original problem. Input, output, databases, forms, codification schemes and processing specifications are drawn up in detail. In the design stage, the programming language and the hardware and software platform in which the new system will run are also decided. There are several tools and techniques used for describing the system design of the system.

These tools and techniques are:
   i. Flowchart
  ii. Data flow diagram (DFD)
 iii. Data dictionary
  iv. Structured English
   v. Decision table
  vi. Decision tree

Each of the above tools for designing will be discussed in detailed in the next lesson.

The system design involves:
   i. Defining precisely the required system output
  ii. Determining the data requirement for producing the output
 iii. Determining the medium and format of files and databases
  iv. Devising processing methods and use of software to produce output
   v. Determine the methods of data capture and data input
  vi. Designing input forms
 vii. Designing codification schemes
viii. Detailed manual procedures
  ix. Documenting the design.

Data Flow Diagram

A data flow diagram (DFD) maps out the flow of information for any development. It mainly uses defined symbols like rectangles, circles and arrows, text labels, to show inputs, outputs, storage points and the routes between each destination. Data Flowcharts can range from simple, even hand-drawn process overviews, to in-depth, multi-level DFDs that dig progressively deeper into how the data is handled. They can be used to analyze an existing system or model a new one. Like all the best diagrams and charts, a DFD can often visually 'say' things that would be hard to explain in words, and they work for both technical and nontechnical audiences, from developer to CEO. That's why DFDs remain so popular after all these years. While they work well for data flow software and systems, they are less applicable nowadays to visualizing interactive, real-time or database-oriented software or systems.

Symbols and Notations Used in DFDs

Using any convention's DFD rules or guidelines, the symbols depict the four components of data flow diagrams.

   1. **External entity:** An external entity is an outside system that sends or receives data. They are the sources and destinations of information that enters or leaves the system. They might be an outside organization or person, a computer system or a business system. They can also be called terminators, sources and sinks or actors. They are typically drawn on the edges of the diagram (Fig. 2.1).

   2. **Process:** A process takes the input and changes the data to produce an output. It might perform computations, or sort data based on logic, or direct the data flow based on business rules. A short label is used to describe the process.

Notation	Yourdon and coad	Gane and sarson
External entity	▭	▭
Process	◯	▢
Data store	⊏	⊏
Data flow	⟶	⟶

Fig. 2.1: Symbols and notations used in DFDs

3. **Data store:** Records or files that hold information for later use, e.g. a database table or a membership forms. Each data store receives a simple label.
4. **Data flow:** It is the route that data takes between the external entities, processes and data stores. It acts as the interface between the other components and is shown with arrows.

Rules of Data Flow Diagram

There are some of the rules while DFD is diagrammed and are:
   i. Each process should have at least one input and an output.
   ii. Each data store should have at least one data flow in and one data flow out.
   iii. Data stored in a system must go through a process.
   iv. All processes in a DFD go to another process or a data store.

DFD Levels and Layers

DFD levels are numbered 0, 1 or 2, and occasionally go to even Level 3 or beyond. The necessary level of detail depends on the scope of what you are trying to accomplish.
   i. DFD Level 0 is also called a Context Diagram. It is a basic overview of the whole system or process being analyzed or modeled. It is designed to be an at-a-glance view, showing the system as a single high-level process, with its relationship to external entities. It should be easily understood by a wide audience, including stakeholders, business analysts, data analysts and developers.
   ii. DFD Level 1 provides a more detailed breakout of pieces of the Context Level Diagram. You will highlight the main functions carried out by the system, as you breakdown the high-level process of the Context Diagram into its subprocesses.
   iii. DFD Level 2 then goes one step deeper into parts of Level 1. It may require more text to reach the necessary level of detail about the system's functioning.

Progression to Levels 3, 4 and beyond is possible, but going beyond Level 3 is uncommon. Doing so can create complexity that makes it difficult to communicate, compare or model effectively.

Using DFD layers, the cascading levels can be nested directly in the diagram, providing a cleaner look with easy access to the deeper dive.

By becoming sufficiently detailed in the DFD, developers and designers can use it to write pseudocode, which is a combination of English and the coding language. Pseudocode facilitates the development of the actual code.

Process Specification

A process specification is a method used to document, analyze and explain the decision-making logic and formulas used to create output data from process input data. Its objective is to flow down and specify regulatory/engineering requirements and procedures. High-quality, consistent data requires clear and complete process specifications.

A process specification reduces ambiguity, allowing an individual or organization to obtain a precise description of executed tasks and accomplishments and validate system design, including the data dictionary and data flow diagrams.

Process specifications are created for primitive processes and data flow diagram processes of a higher level (minispecs). Process logic is best represented through structured English, decision tables, decision trees or specified formulas or algorithms and is used to communicate engineering requirements and procedures to businesses involved in the creation of a process. Process descriptions may exist on a form or in a computer aided software engineering (CASE) tool repository.

Process specifications are not created for processes requiring physical input or output, processes representing simple data validation or processes with pre-existing and prewritten code.

Input/Output Design

Input Design

In an information system, input is the raw data that is processed to produce output. During the input design, the developers must consider the input devices, such as PC, MICR, OMR, etc.

Therefore, the quality of system input determines the quality of system output. Well-designed input forms and screens have following properties:

    i. It should serve specific purpose effectively such as storing, recording, and retrieving the information.
    ii. It ensures proper completion with accuracy.
    iii. It should be easy to fill and straightforward.
    iv. It should focus on user's attention, consistency, and simplicity.

All these objectives are obtained using the knowledge of basic design principles regarding:

    a. What are the inputs needed for the system?
    b. How end users respond to different elements of forms and screens.

Objectives for Input Design

The objectives of input design are:

    i. To design data entry and input procedures
    ii. To reduce input volume
    iii. To design source documents for data capture or devise other data capture methods

iv. To design input data records, data entry screens, user interface screens, etc.

v. To use validation checks and develop effective input controls.

Data Input Methods

It is important to design appropriate data input methods to prevent errors while entering data. These methods depend on whether the data is entered by customers in forms manually and later entered by data entry operators, or data is directly entered by users on the PCs.

A system should prevent user from making mistakes by:

i. Clear form design by leaving enough space for writing legibly.

ii. Clear instructions to fill form.

iii. Clear form design.

iv. Reducing key strokes.

v. Immediate error feedback.

Some of the popular data input methods are:

i. Batch input method (offline data input method)

ii. Online data input method

iii. Computer readable forms

iv. Interactive data input

Input Integrity Controls

Input integrity controls include a number of methods to eliminate common input errors by end-users. They also include checks on the value of individual fields; both for format and the completeness of all inputs.

Audit trails for data entry and other system operations are created using transaction logs which gives a record of all changes introduced in the database to provide security and means of recovery in case of any failure.

Output Design

The design of output is the most important task of any system. During output design, developers identify the type of outputs needed, and consider the necessary output controls and prototype report layouts.

Objectives of Output Design

The objectives of input design are:

i. To develop output design that serves the intended purpose and eliminates the production of unwanted output.

ii. To develop the output design that meets the end users requirements.

iii. To deliver the appropriate quantity of output.

iv. To form the output in appropriate format and direct it to the right person.

v. To make the output available on time for making good decisions.

Let us now go through various types of outputs

External Outputs

Manufacturers create and design external outputs for printers. External outputs enable the system to leave the trigger actions on the part of their recipients or confirm actions to their recipients.

Some of the external outputs are designed as turnaround outputs, which are implemented as a form and re-enter the system as an input.

Internal Outputs

Internal outputs are present inside the system, and used by end-users and managers. They support the management in decision-making and reporting.

There are three types of reports produced by management information:

1. **Detailed reports:** They contain present information which has almost no filtering or restriction generated to assist management planning and control.
2. **Summary reports:** They contain trends and potential problems which are categorized and summarized that are generated for managers who do not want details.
3. **Exception reports:** They contain exceptions, filtered data to some condition or standard before presenting it to the manager, as information.

Output Integrity Controls

Output integrity controls include routing codes to identify the receiving system, and verification messages to confirm successful receipt of messages that are handled by network protocol.

Printed or screen-format reports should include a date/time for report printing and the data. Multipage reports contain report title or description, and pagination. Pre-printed forms usually include a version number and effective date.

Process Life Cycle

A process changes its state during its execution which is called the **process life cycle**. A process life cycle consists of five stages which are (Fig. 2.2 & Table 2.1)

   i. New
  ii. Running
 iii. Waiting

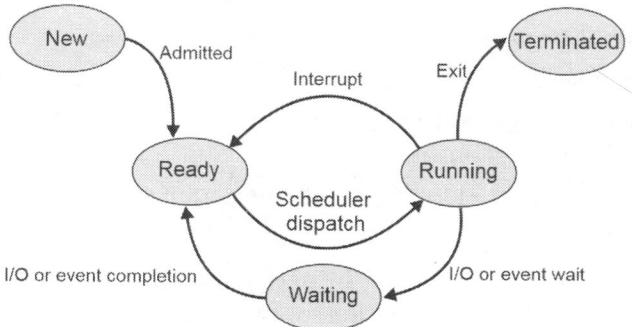

Fig. 2.2: Process life cycle

iv. Ready

v. Terminated.

Table 2.1: Process life cycles

Stages	Description
New	The process which is being created
Running	Instructions being executed
Waiting	The process is waiting for an event to get occur
Ready	The process is waiting to be assigned to a processor
Terminated	The process completed its execution

These names of the states are uninformed and they vary across operating system. These states are mostly found on all systems but some operating systems also more finely define process states. Processer can hold only one process at a time simply it can be running one process at a time. However, many processes may be ready or waiting.

Planning and Managing the Project

Project planning is at the heart of the project life cycle, and tells everyone involved where you're going and how you're going to get there. The planning phase is when the project plans are documented, the project deliverables and requirements are defined, and the project schedule is created. It involves creating a set of plans to help guide your team through the implementation and closure phases of the project. The plans created during this phase will help you manage time, cost, quality, changes, risk, and related issues. They will also help you control staff and external suppliers to ensure that you deliver the project on time, within budget, and within schedule.

The project planning phase is often the most challenging phase for a project manager, as you need to make an educated guess about the staff, resources, and equipment needed to complete your project. You may also need to plan your communications and procurement activities, as well as contract any third-party suppliers.

The purpose of the project planning phase is to:

i. Establish business requirements

ii. Establish cost, schedule, list of deliverables, and delivery dates

iii. Establish resources plans

iv. Obtain management approval and proceed to the next phase.

The basic processes of project planning are:

1. **Scope planning:** Specifying the in-scope requirements for the project to facilitate creating the work breakdown structure.

2. **Preparation of the work breakdown structure:** Spelling out the breakdown of the project into tasks and sub-tasks.

3. **Project schedule development:** Listing the entire schedule of the activities and detailing their sequence of implementation.

4. **Resource planning:** Indicating who will do what work, at which time, and if any special skills are needed to accomplish the project tasks.

5. **Budget planning:** Specifying the budgeted cost to be incurred at the completion of the project.

6. **Procurement planning:** Focusing on vendors outside your company and subcontracting.

7. **Risk management:** Planning for possible risks and considering optional contingency plans and mitigation strategies.

8. **Quality planning:** Assessing quality criteria to be used for the project.

9. **Communication planning:** Designing the communication strategy with all project stakeholders.

The planning phase refines the project's objectives, which were gathered during the initiation phase. It includes planning the steps necessary to meet those objectives by further identifying the specific activities and resources required to complete the project. Now that these objectives have been recognized, they must be clearly articulated, detailing an in-depth scrutiny of each recognized objective. With such scrutiny, our understanding of the objective may change. Often the very act of trying to describe something precisely gives us a better understanding of what we are looking at. This articulation serves as the basis for the development of requirements. What this means is that after an objective has been clearly articulated, we can describe it in concrete (measurable) terms and identify what we have to do to achieve it. Obviously, if we do a poor job of articulating the objective, our requirements will be misdirected and the resulting project will not represent the true need.

Example: A web user may ask for a fast system. The quantitative requirement should be all screens must load in under three seconds. Describing the time limit during which the screen must load is specific and tangible. For that reason, you'll know that the requirement has been successfully completed when the objective has been met.

ISOLATED KEY POINTS

Data and Information

In data and information; data is the plural of the word datum, mean facts and may be looked upon as the raw materials for information. The term information cannot be precisely defined as it has some abstract meaning. Information can be exchanged between different sources which are capable of understanding those. Information enriches the knowledge of human being and helps to achieve the specific purpose. In the perspective of computer science, we shall say that information is data arranged in a relevant order to fulfill the necessity of the problems concerned. Information may be represented by combinations of symbols which may be alphabetic or numeric or both, i.e. alphanumeric.

System Design

System design is the phase that bridges the gap between problem domain and the existing system in a manageable way. This phase focuses on the solution domain, i.e. "how to implement?"

It is the phase where the SRS document is converted into a format that can be implemented and decides how the system will operate.

In this phase, the complex activity of system development is divided into several smaller sub-activities, which coordinate with each other to achieve the main objective of system development.

Inputs to System Design

System design takes the following inputs:

- Statement of work
- Requirement determination plan
- Current situation analysis
- Proposed system requirements including a conceptual data model, modified DFDs, and Metadata (data about data).

Outputs for System Design

System design gives the following outputs:

- Infrastructure and organizational changes for the proposed system.
- A data schema, often a relational schema.
- Metadata to define the tables/files and columns/data-items.
- A function hierarchy diagram or web page map that graphically describes the program structure.
- Actual or pseudocode for each module in the program.
- A prototype for the proposed system.

Types of System Design

Logical Design

Logical design pertains to an abstract representation of the data flow, inputs, and outputs of the system. It describes the inputs (sources), outputs (destinations), databases (data stores), procedures (data flows) all in a format that meets the user requirements.

While preparing the logical design of a system, the system analyst specifies the user needs at level of detail that virtually determines the information flow into and out of the system and the required data sources. Data flow diagram, E-R diagram modeling are used.

Physical Design

Physical design relates to the actual input and output processes of the system. It focuses on how data is entered into a system, verified, processed, and displayed as output.

It produces the working system by defining the design specification that specifies exactly what the candidate system does. It is concerned with user interface design, process design, and data design.

Architectural Design

It is also known as high level design that focuses on the design of system architecture. It describes the structure and behavior of the system. It defines the structure and relationship between various modules of system development process.

Detailed Design

It follows architectural design and focuses on development of each module.

Conceptual Data Modeling

It is representation of organizational data which includes all the major entities and relationship. System analysts develop a conceptual data model for the current system that supports the scope and requirement for the proposed system.

PRACTICE QUESTIONS

Long Answer Type Questions

1. What is the difference between data and information?
2. Explain the various symbol and notations used in DFD.
3. Differentiate between decision table and decision tree.
4. Explain the basic principles of project planning.
5. What is process life cycle? Explain with diagram.

OBJECTIVE TYPE QUESTIONS

1. A DFD provides no information about the timing or ordering of processes, or about whether processes will operate in sequence or in parallel.
   a. True
   b. False

2. The first component of the DFD is known as a _____ common synonyms are a bubble, a function, or a transformation.
   a. Flow
   b. Process
   c. Square
   d. Entity

3. Initially a context diagram is drawn, which is a simple representation of the entire system under investigation. This is followed by a Level 1 diagram
   a. Level 0 diagram
   b. Level 1 diagram
   c. Level A diagram
   d. Both A and B

4. Context diagram defines the scope of the system by identifying the system boundary:
   a. Context diagram
   b. Level 0 DFD
   c. Level 1 DFD
   d. Level 2 DFD

5. A _____ is represented graphically by an arrow into or out of a process
   a. Process
   b. Entity
   c. Level
   d. Flow

6. Composite data flow on one level can be split into its component data flows on the next level-but new data cannot be added and all data in the composite must be included in the sub-flows
   a. True
   b. False

7. **A data flow may or may not be attached to at least one process**
   a. True
   b. False

8. _____ **is to organize the overall DFD in a series of levels so that each level provides successively more detail about a portion of the level above it.**
   a. Split DFDs
   b. Leveled DFDs
   c. Flow DFDs
   d. All of Above

9. **Objects in a set of DFDs have unique names**
   a. True
   b. False

10. **Lowest level DFDs may add new data flows to represent exception handling, i.e. error messages**
    a. True
    b. False

11. **A _____ is a decision support tool that uses a tree-like graph or model of decisions and their possible consequences, including chance event outcomes, resource costs, and utility.**
    a. Decision tree
    b. Graphs
    c. Trees
    d. Neural Networks

12. **Decision tree is a display of an algorithm.**
    a. True
    b. False

ANSWERS KEY					
1. a	2. b	3. b	4. a	5. d	6. a
7. b	8. b	9. a	10. a	11. a	12. a

Web Technologies

INTERNET

The Internet is a global wide area network that connects computer systems across the world. The Internet is sometimes called simply 'the Net,' is a worldwide system of computer networks, a network of networks in which users at anyone computer can, if they have permission, get information from any other computer (and sometimes talk directly to users at other computers).

In order to connect to the Internet, you must have access to an Internet service provider (ISP), which acts the middleman between you and the Internet.

The Internet provides different online services. Some examples include:

1. **Web:** A collection of billions of webpages that you can view with a web browser
2. **Email:** The most common method of sending and receiving messages online
3. **Social media:** Websites and apps that allow people to share comments, photos, and videos
4. **Online gaming:** Games that allow people to play with and against each other over the Internet
5. **Software updates:** Operating system and application updates can typically downloaded from the Internet.

Concept of WWW

WWW: The World Wide Web, abbreviated as WWW and commonly known as the Web, is a system of interlinked hypertext documents accessed via the Internet. With a web browser, one can view web pages that may contain text, images, videos, and other multimedia and navigate between them via hyperlinks.

1. WWW is stands for World Wide Web.
2. The World Wide Web (WWW) is a global information medium which users can read and write via computer connected to the internet.
3. The Web, or World Wide Web, is basically a system of Internet servers that support specially formatted documents. The documents are formatted in a markup language called HTML (Hypertext Markup Language) that supports links to other documents, as well as graphics, audio, and video files.
4. In short, World Wide Web (WWW) is collection of text pages, digital photographs, music files, videos, and animations you can access over the Internet.

5. Web pages are primarily text documents formatted and annotated with Hypertext Markup Language (HTML). In addition to formatted text, web pages may contain images, video, and software components that are rendered in the user's web browser as coherent pages of multimedia content.

6. The terms Internet and World Wide Web are often used without much distinction. However, the two are not the same.

7. The Internet is a global system of interconnected computer networks. In contrast, the World Wide Web is one of the services transferred over these networks. It is a collection of text documents and other resources, linked by hyperlinks and URLs, usually accessed by web browsers, from web servers.

8. There are several applications called Web browsers that make it easy to access the World Wide Web, e.g. Firefox, Microsoft's Internet Explorer, Chrome, etc.

9. Users access the World Wide Web facilities via a client called a browser, which provides transparent access to the WWW servers. User can access WWW via two way such us:

History of WWW

Tim Berners-Lee, in 1980 was investigating how computer could store information with random links. In 1989, while working at European Particle Physics Laboratory, he proposed to idea of global hypertext space in which any network-accessible information could be referred to by single "universal Document Identifier". After that in 1990, this idea expanded with further program and knows as World Wide Web.

Internet and WWW

The Internet, linking your computer to other computers around the world, is a way of transporting content. The Web is software that lets you use that content...or contribute your own. The Web, running on the mostly invisible Internet, is what you see and click on in your computer's browser.

The Internet is infrastructure while the Web is service on top of that infrastructure. The Internet is a global network of networks while the Web, also referred formally as World Wide Web (www) is collection of information which is accessed via the Internet. Alternatively, the Internet can be viewed as a big book-store while the Web can be viewed as collection of books on that store.

What is Website?

A website is normally built around a central page, called a welcome page, which offers links to a group of other pages hosted on the same server, and sometimes 'external' links, which lead to pages hosted by another server.

Web technologies are a general terms referring to the many languages and multimedia packages that are used in conjunction with one another, to produce dynamic web sites. Computers do not communicate with each other the way that people do. Instead, computers require codes, or directions. These binary codes and commands allow computers to process needed information. The methods by which computers communicate with each other through the use of markup languages and multimedia packages is known as web technology.

Introduction of HTML

HTML stands for Hyper Text Markup Language. It is used to design web pages using markup language. HTML is the combination of Hypertext and Markup language. Hypertext defines the link between the web pages. Markup language is used to define the text document within tag which defines the structure of web pages. This language is used to annotate (make notes for the computer) text so that a machine can understand it and manipulate text accordingly. Most of markup (e.g. HTML) languages are human readable. Language uses tags to define what manipulation has to be done on the text.

What is HTML?

a. Stands for Hypertext Markup Language.

b. Most documents that appear on the World Wide Web were written in HTML.

c. HTML is a markup language, not a programming language. In fact, the term HTML is an acronym that stands for Hypertext Markup Language.

d. We can apply this markup language to your pages to display text, images, sound and movie files, and almost any other type of electronic information.

e. We use the language to format documents and link them together, regardless of the type of computer with which the file was originally created.

HTML history: HTML was created by Tim Berners-Lee in 1991. The first ever version of HTML was HTML 1.0 but the first standard version was HTML 2.0 which was published in 1999. HTML is a markup language which is used by the browser to manipulate text, images and other content to display it in required format.

HTML planning for designing web pages: Breaking Up Your Content into Main Topics With your goals in mind, try to organize your content into main topics or sections, chunking related information together under a single topic. Ideas for Organization and Navigation At this point, you should have a good idea of what you want to talk about as well as a list of topics. The next step is to actually start structuring the information you have into a set of web pages. Before you do that, however, consider some standard structures that have been used in other help systems and online tools. This section describes some of these structures, their various features, some important considerations, including the following.

Model and structure of a Web site: You need to know what the following terms mean and how they apply to the body of work you're developing for the Web.

Website: A collection of one or more web pages linked together in a meaningful way that, as a whole, describes a body of information or creates an overall effect.

Web server: A computer on the Internet or an intranet that delivers Web pages and other files in response to browser requests.

Web page: A single document on a website, usually consisting of an HTML document and any items that are displayed within that document such as inline images.

Home page: The entry page for a website, which can link to additional pages on the same website or pages on other sites.

Developing websites: Designing a website, like designing a book outline, a building plan, or a painting, can sometimes be a complex and involved process.

Having a plan before you begin can help you keep the details straight and help you develop the finished product with fewer false starts. Today, you learned how to put together a simple plan and structure for creating a set of web pages, including the following:

a. Deciding what sort of content to present

b. Coming up with a set of goals for that content

c. Deciding on a set of topics

d. Organizing and storyboarding the website basic.

HTML Elements

1. An element consists of three basic parts: an opening tag, the element's content, and finally, a closing tag.

   <p> - opening paragraph tag Element

   Content - paragraph words

   </p> - closing tag

2. Every (web) page requires four critical elements: the html, head, title, and body elements.

   <html> Element...</html>

   a. <html> begins and ends each and every web page.

   b. Its purpose is to encapsulate all the HTML code and describe the HTML document to the web browser.

   <html></html>

   <head> Element

   c. The <head> element is "next" as they say. As long as it falls somewhere between your <html> tag and your web page content (<body>).

   d. The head functions "behind the scenes." Tags placed within the head element are not directly displayed by web browsers.

   e. We will be placing the <title> element here.

   f. Other elements used for scripting (JavaScript) and formatting (CSS) will eventually be introduced and you will have to place them within your head element.

   <html>

   <head>

   </head>

   </html>

   The <title> Element

   g. Place the <title> tag within the <head> element to title your page.

   h. The words you write between the opening and closing <title></title> tags will be displayed at the top of a viewer's browser.

   <html><head><title>My WebPage!</title></head></html>

   The <body> Element

   i. The <body> element is where all content is placed. (Paragraphs, pictures, tables, etc).

j. The body element will encapsulate all of your webpage's viewable content.
```
<html>
<head><title>My WebPage!</title></head>
<body>
Hello World! All my content goes here!
</body>
</html>
```

HTML Tags

a. A web browser reads an HTML document top to bottom, left to right.
b. Each time the browser finds a tag, it is displayed accordingly (paragraphs look like paragraphs, tables look like tables, etc).
c. Tags have 3 major parts—opening tag(s), content(s), and closing tag(s).
d. Recall that a completed tag is termed an element.

1. Paragraph Tag <p>

a. The <p> tag defines a paragraph. Using this tag places a blank line above and below the text of the paragraph.
b. <p>Avoid losing floppy disks with important school...</p>
c. <p>For instance, let's say you had a HUGE school...</p>

2. HTML—headings 1:6

a. A heading in HTML is just what we might expect, a title or subtitle.
b. By placing text inside of <h1> (heading) tags, the text displays bold and the size of the text depends on the number of heading (1–6).
c. Headings are numbered 1–6, with 1 being the largest heading and 6 being the smallest.
```
<html><body>
<h1>This is heading 1</h1><h2>This is heading 2</h2><h3>This is heading 3</h3>
<h4>This is heading 4</h4><h5>This is heading 5</h5><h6>This is heading 6</h6>
</body></html>
```

3. Line breaks

a. Line breaks are different then most of the tags we have seen so far. A line break ends the line you are currently on and resumes on the next line.
b. <p>Darshan
 Computer
</p>

HTML Lists

There are three different types of lists.

A <ol> tag starts an ordered list, <ul> for unordered lists, and <dl> for definition lists.

a. <ul> - unordered list; bullets
b. <ol> - ordered list; numbers
c. <dl> - definition list; dictionary

1. HTML ordered lists

a. Use the <ol> tag to begin an ordered list. Place the <li> (list item) tag between your opening <ol> and closing </ol> tags to create list items.

b. Ordered simply means numbered, as the list below demonstrates.

```
<ol>
<li>Find a Job</li>
<li>Move Out</li>
</ol>
<li>Get a Degree</li>
</ol>
```

c. **There are four other types of ordered lists.** Instead of generic numbers you can replace them with Roman numerals or letters, both capital and lowercase. Use the type attribute to change the numbering.

```
<oltype="a">
<oltype="A">
<oltype="i">
<ol type="I">
</ol>
```

2. HTML unordered lists

a. Create a bulleted list with the <ul> tag. The bullet itself comes in three subtypes: squares, discs, and circles.

b. The default bullet displayed by most web browsers is the traditional full disc.

```
<ul>
<li>Milk</li>
<li>Chocolate</li>
</ul>
```

c. There are three other types of unordered lists.

```
<oltype="square">
<ol type="disc">
<oltype="circle">
</ol>
```

3. HTML definition term lists

Make definition lists as seen in dictionaries using the <dl> tag. These lists displace the term word just above the definition itself for a unique look. It is

```
<dl>
<dt><b>Fromage</b></dt>
<dd>French word for cheese.</dd>
<dt><b>Voiture</b></dt>
<dd>French word for car.</dd>
</dl>
```

HTML—Formatting Elements

Several tags exist to further amplify text elements. These formatting tags can make text bold, italic, sub/superscripted, and more (Table 3.1).

Table 3.1: HTML—formatting elements

Tag	Description	Example
<b>	The <b> tag specifies bold text.	<b>Bold Text</b>
<i>	The <i> tag specifies italic text.	<i>Italic Text</i>
<em>	The<em> tag specifies emphasis text	<em>Emphasized Text</em>
<sup>	The <sup> tag defines superscript text. Superscript text appears half a character above the baseline. Superscript text can be used for footnotes, like WWW.	<p>This text contains^{superscript}text.</p>
<sub>	The <sub> tag defines subscript text. Subscript text appears half a character below the baseline. Subscript text can be used for chemical formulas, like H_2O.	<p>An example of _{subscripted Text}</p>
<tt>	The <tt> tag defines teletype text.	<p><tt>This text is Teletype text.</tt></p>
<blink>	The <blink> tag is used for blinking the text.	<blink> blinking text tag</blink>

HTML Color Coding System—Color Names

There are three different methods to set color.
We can set color using three methods.

a. Using color name

       <body bgcolor="red">
       <font color="red">
       <body bgcolor="rgb(72,0,0)">
       <font color="rgb(72,0,0)">

b. Using hexadecimal value

       <body bgcolor="#ffff00">
       <font color="#ffff00">

The target attribute defines whether to open the page in a separate window, or to open the link in the current browser window (Table 3.2).

Table 3.2: HTML color coding system

	HTML code
target=" _blank"	Opens new page in a new browser window
target=" _self"	Loads the new page in current window
target=" _parent"	Loads new page into a frame that is superior to where the link lies
target=" _top"	Loads new page into the current browser window, cancelling all frames

Anchors

a. To link to sections of your existing page a name must be given to the anchor.

b. In the example below, we've created a mini Table of contents for this page.

c. By placing blank anchors just after each heading, and naming them, we can then create reference links to those sections on this page as shown below.

d. First, the headings of this page contain blank, named anchors. They look like this.

```
<h2>HTML Links and Anchors<a name="top"></a></h2>
<h2>HTML Text Links<a name="text"></a></h2>
<h2>HTML Email<a name="email"></a></h2>
```

e. Now create the reference links, placing the # symbol followed by the name of the anchor in the href of the new link.

```
<a href="#top">Go to the Top</a>
<a href="#text">Learn about Text Links</a>
<a href="#email">Learn about Email Links</a>
```

HTML—Images

Use the <img /> tag to place an image on your web page.

```
<imgsrc="sunset.gif" />
```

1. Image src

a. Above we have defined the src attribute.

b. Src stands for source, the source of the image or more appropriately, where the picture file is located.

c. There are two ways to define the source of an image. First you may use a standard URL. (src=http://www.Xyz.com/pics/htmlT/sunset.gif) As your second choice, you may copy or upload the file onto your web server and access it locally using standard directory tree methods. (src="../sunset.gif")

d. The location of this picture file is in relation to your location of your .html file (Table 3.3).

e. A URL cannot contain drive letters

f. Therefore something like src="C:\\www\web\pics\" will not work. Pictures must be uploaded along with your .html file to your web server.

2. Alternative attribute

The alt attribute specifies alternate text to be displayed if for some reason the browser cannot find the image, or if a user has image files disabled.

```
<imgsrc="http://example.com/brokenlink/sunset.gif" alt="Beautiful Sunset" />
```

Table 3.3: HTML URL types

URL types	
Local Src	Location description
src="sunset.gif"	picture file resides in same directory as .html file
src="../sunset.gif"	picture file resides in previous directory as .html file
src="../pics/sunset.gif"	picture file resides in the pic directory in a previous directory as .html file

3. Image height and width

To define the height and width of the image, rather than letting the browser compute the size, use the height and width attributes.

```
<imgsrc="sunset.gif" height="50" width="100">
```

4. Vertically and horizontally align images

a. Use the align and valign attributes to place images within your body, tables, or sections.

1. Align (Horizontal)

1. Right 2. left 3. center

2. Valign (Vertical)

1. Top 2. bottom 3. center

b. Below is an example of how to align an image to the right of a paragraph

```
<p>This is paragraph 1, yes it is...</p>
```

```
<p><imgsrc="sunset.gif" align="right">The image will appear along the...isn't it? </p>
```

5. Images as links

Images are very useful for links and can be created with the HTML below.

```
<a href="http://www.xyz.com/"><imgsrc="sunset.gif"></a>
```

HTML Forms

A form will take input from the viewer and depending on your needs, you may store that data into a file, place an order, gather user statistics, register the person to your web forum, or maybe subscribe them to your weekly newsletter.

Making a Form

<form> is main tag to build a form.

It has a few optional attributes too. Below is an example of the form element.

```
<form action="processform.php" method="post">
```

```
</form>
```

The action attribute tells the HTML where to send the collected information, while the method attribute describes the way to send it.

Type of Input

a. The main tag for collecting information from the user is <input>.

b. The tag itself contains a name attribute, so that we can refer to the input by a name, and the size of the entry box in characters.

c. There are quite few different types of input to choose from:

d. <input type="text"/> this is the default input type and accepts characters and numbers into a text box. It can also have a value attribute attached to it, which will give it an initial value.

e. <input type="password"/> this is similar to the above text box but anything that is typed cannot be seen; instead an asterisk is printed to cover up the entry. As the name suggests, this is used for password entry.

f. <input type="checkbox"/> this gives a box that can be toggled between checked and unchecked. It can initially be set to one or the other with checked="checked".

g. <input type="radio"/> this is similar to checkbox but in group of radio buttons only one can be selected at a time. This can also have an initial checked state on one of the radio buttons.

h. <input type="file"/>This will give a box to allow you to choose a file similar to when you open or save files usually on your machine. It can be used to select a file on the local machine for upload to a server.

i. <input type="submit"/> this allows a form to be submitted. When pressed, the information will be passed on for processing, usually to a script mentioned in the action attribute option of the form.

j. <input type="image"/> this will also submit the form when selected and, like the img tag, requires the src attribute to specify an associated image.

k. <input type="button"/> this makes a button available.

l. <input type="reset"/> this will reset the form to its initial state when selected.

m. <input type="hidden"/> this allows hidden data (not seen by the user) to be passed along with the form.

HTML Text Fields

The <input> has a few attributes that you should be aware of.

Type—determines what kind of input field it will be. Possible choices are text, submit, and password.

Name—assigns a name to the given field so that you may reference it later.

Size—sets the horizontal width of the field. The unit of measurement is in blank spaces.

Maxlength—dictates the maximum number of characters that can be entered.

<form method="post" action="mailto:youremail@email.com">

Name: <input type="text" size="10" maxlength="40" name="name">

Password: <input type="password" size="10" maxlength="10" name="password">

HTML Radio Buttons

Radio buttons are a popular form of interaction. You may have seen them on quizzes, questionnaires, and other web sites that give the user a multiple choice question. that relate to the radio button.

<form method="post" action="mailto:youremail@email.com"> What kind of shirt are you wearing?

Shade:

<input type="radio" name="shade" value="dark">Dark

<input type="radio" name="shade" value="light">Light

</form>

HTML Check Boxes

Check boxes allow for multiple items to be selected for a certain group of choices. The check box's name and value attributes behave the same as a radio button.

```
<form method="post" action="mailto:youremail@email.com"> Select your favorite
```
cartoon characters.
```
<input type="checkbox" name="toon" value="Goofy">Goofy
<input type="checkbox" name="toon" value="Donald">Donald
<input type="checkbox" name="toon" value="Bugs">Bugs Bunny
</form>
```

HTML Text Areas

Text areas serve as an input field for viewers to place their own comments onto forums and the like use text areas to post what you type onto their site using scripts. For this form, the text area is used as a way to write comments to somebody.

Rows and columns need to be specified as attributes to the <textarea> tag.

HTML Tables

The <table> tag is used to begin a table. Within a table element are the <tr> (table rows) and

```
<td> (table columns) tags.
    <table border="1">
    <tr><td>Row 1 Cell 1</td><td>Row 1 Cell 2</td></tr>
    <tr><td>Row 2 Cell 1</td><td>Row 2 Cell 2</td></tr>
    </table>
```

Table 3.4: HTML Table	
Row 1 Cell 1	Row 1 Cell 2
Row 2 Cell 1	Row 2 Cell 2

Content is placed within tables cells. A table cell is defined by <td> and </td>. The border attribute defines how wide the table's border will be.

Spanning Multiple Rows and Cells

Use rowspan to span multiple rows and colspan to span multiple columns.

Note: If you would like to place headers at the top of your columns, use the <th> tag as shown below. By default these headers are bold to set them apart from the rest of your table's content.

```
<table border="1"><tr><th>Column 1</th><th>Column 2</th><th>Column 3</th></tr>
<tr><td rowspan="2">Row 1 Cell 1</td><td>Row 1 Cell 2</td><td>Row 1 Cell 3</td></tr>
<tr><td>Row 2 Cell 2</td><td>Row 2 Cell 3</td></tr>
<tr><td colspan="3">Row 3 Cell 1</td></tr>
</table>
```

Table 3.5: Spanning multiple rows and cells		
Column 1	*Column 2*	*Column 3*
Row 1 Cell 1	Row 1 Cell 2	Row 1 Cell 3
	Row 2 Cell 2	Row 2 Cell 3
Row 3 Cell 1		

Cell Padding and Spacing

a. With the cell padding and cell spacing attributes you will be able to adjust the white space on your tables. Spacing defines the width of the border, while padding represents the distance between cell borders and the content within. Color has been added to the table to emphasize these attributes (Table 3.6).

```
<table border="1" cell spacing="10" bgcolor="rgb(0,255,0)">
<tr><th>Column 1</th><th>Column 2</th></tr>
<tr><td>Row 1 Cell 1</td><td>Row 1 Cell 2</td></tr>
<tr><td>Row 2 Cell 1</td><td>Row 2 Cell 2</td></tr>
</table>
```

Table 3.6: Cell padding and spacing	
Column 1	*Column 2*
Row 1 Cell 1	Row 1 Cell 2
Row 2 Cell 1	Row 2 Cell 2

And now we will change the cell padding of the table and remove the cell spacing from the previous example.

```
<table border="1" cell padding="10" bgcolor="rgb(0,255,0)">
<tr><th>Column 1</th><th>Column 2</th></tr>
<tr><td>Row 1 Cell 1</td><td>Row 1 Cell 2</td></tr>
<tr><td>Row 2 Cell 1</td><td>Row 2 Cell 2</td></tr>
</table>
```

Table 3.7: Cell padding and spacing	
Column 1	*Column 2*
Row 1 Cell 1	Row 1 Cell 2
Row 2 Cell 1	Row 2 Cell 2

HTML - <!— Comments —>

a. A comment is a way for you as the web page developer to control what lines of code are to be ignored by the web browser.

b. Comment syntax may be a little complicated, there is an opening and a closing much like tags.

1. <!— Opening comment
2. — > Closing comment

<!—Note to self: This is my banner image! Don't forget —>

<imgsrc="http://www.website.com/pics/anyimage.jpg" height="100" width="200"/>

Introduction to HTML5

The DOCTYPE declaration for HTML5 is very simple:

<!DOCTYPE html>

The character encoding (charset) declaration is also very simple:

<meta charset="UTF-8">

New HTML5 elements:

a. New semantic elements like <header>, <footer>, <article>, and <section>.

b. New form control attributes like number, date, time, calendar, and range.

c. New graphic elements: <svg> and <canvas>.

d. New multimedia elements: <audio> and <video>.

e. Elements Removed in HTML5

The following HTML4 elements have been removed from HTML5:

Table 3.8: HTML5

Element	Use instead
<acronym>	<abbr>
<applet>	<object>
<basefont>	CSS
<big>	CSS
<center>	CSS
<dir>	<ul>
<font>	CSS
<frame>	
<frameset>	
<noframes>	
<strike>	CSS
<tt>	CSS

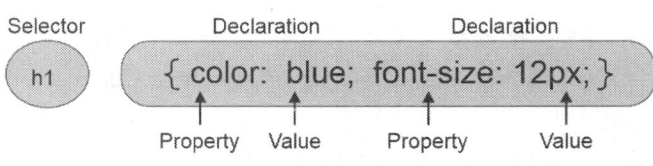

Fig. 3.1: HTML5

XML

What is XML?

1. XML is a meta-language, which can be used to store data and act as a mechanism to transfer information between dissimilar systems.
2. XML stands for EXtensible Markup Language.
3. XML is a markup language much like HTML.
4. XML was designed to describe data.
5. XML tags are not predefined in XML. You must define your own tags.
6. XML is self describing.
7. XML uses a DTD (Document Type Definition) to formally describe the data.

```
<?xml version="1.0"?>
<Person>
<Firstname>Ralph</Firstname>
<Lastname>Mosely</Lastname>
</Person>
```

Difference between XML and HTML

Table 3.9: Difference between XML and HTML

XML	HTML
XML was designed to store data and transfer the data	HTML was designed to display data
XML focuses on what data is	HTML focus on how data looks
In XML you can design your own tag	HTML has predefined tags
XML uses parser to check and read xml fileseg. DOM, SAX	HTML don't use any kind of parser

Use of XML

1. Used to exchange data between dissimilar systems.
2. Used to describe content of document.
3. XML can be used as database to store data.

Features of XML

1. XML has its own tag so it's self describing.
2. Language independent: Any language is able to read and write XML.
3. OS independent: Can be work on any platform.
4. Readability: It is a plain text file in user readable format so you can edit or viewin simple editor.
5. Hierarchical: It has hierarchical structure which is powerful to express complex data and simple to understand.

XML Key Component

1. XML root element

XML must have root element. The first element after xml version declaration in file is a root element.

```
<bookstore>
    <book category="CHILDREN">
            <title>Harry Potter</title>
            <author>J K. Rowling</author>
            <year>2005</year>
            <price>29.99</price>
    </book>
</bookstore>
```

In above example <bookstore> is root element.

2. XML element

An XML element is everything from (including) the element's start tag to (including) the element's end tag.

In above example <title>, <author>, <year> and <price> are elements.

3. XML attribute

a. Attributes provide additional information about an element.

b. Attributes often provide information that is not a part of the data. In the example below, the file type is irrelevant to the data, but can be important to the software that wants to manipulate the element

```
<file type="gif">computer.gif</file>
```

c. XML attributes must be quoted

d. Attribute values must always be quoted. Either single or double quotes can be used. For a person's sex, the person element can be written like this:

```
<person sex="female"> or <person sex='female'>
```

4. XML namespace

a. The XML namespace is a special type of reserved XML attribute that you place in an XML tag.

b. The reserved attribute is actually more like a prefix that you attach to any namespace you create.

c. This attribute prefix is "xmlns:" which stands for XML namespace.

d. The colon is used to separate the prefix from your namespace that you are creating.

e. Xmlns must have a unique value that no other namespace in the document has. What is commonly used is the URI (Uniform Resource Identifier) or the more commonly used URL.

Create a XML file that contains Book Information.

```
<xml version="1.0"?>
<bookstore>
  <book>
    <title>Learning XML</title>
    <author>Erik T. Ray</author>
    <year>2003</year>
```

```
    <price>39.95</price>
  </book>
  <book>
    <title>WAD</title>
    <author>Ralph Mosely</author>
    <year>2001</year>
    <price>395</price>
  </book>
</bookstore>
```

Cascading Style Sheets (CSS)

One of the most important aspects of HTML is the capability to separate presentation and content. A style is simply a set of formatting instructions that can be applied to a piece of text. There are three mechanisms by which we can apply styles to our HTML documents.

Inline style sheet: Style can be defined within the basic HTML tag.

Internal style sheet: Style can be defined in the <head> tag.

External style sheet: Styles can be defined in external files called stylesheets which can then be used in any document by including the style sheet via a URL.

What is CSS?

1. CSS stands for cascading style sheets
2. Styles define how to display HTML elements
3. External style sheets can save a lot of work
4. External style sheets are stored in CSS files.

Importance of CSS

1. CSS defines HOW HTML elements are to be displayed.
2. Styles are normally saved in external .css files. External style sheets enable you to change the appearance and layout of all the pages in a Web site, just by editing one single file.

Syntax of CSS

1. A CSS rule has two main parts—a selector, and one or more declarations:
2. The selector is normally the HTML element you want to style.
3. Each declaration consists of a property and a value.
4. The property is the style attribute you want to change. Each property has a value.

There are three ways of inserting a style sheet:

a. External style sheet
b. Internal/embedded style sheet
c. Inline style.

1. External style sheet

a. When using CSS it is preferable to keep the CSS separate from your HTML.

b. Placing CSS in a separate file allows the web designer to completely differentiate between content (HTML) and design (CSS).

c. External CSS is a file that contains only CSS code and is saved with a ".css" file extension.

d. This CSS file is then referenced in your HTML using the <link> instead of <style>.

File creation

a. Open up notepad.exe, or any other plain text editor and type the following CSS code:

body{ background-color: gray;} p { color: blue; }h3{ color: white; }

b. Save the file as a CSS (.css) file.

c. Name the file "test.css" (without the quotes). Now create a new HTML file and fill it with the following code.

```
<html><head>
<link rel="style sheet" type="text/css" href="test.css" /></head>
<body>
<h3> A White Header </h3>
<p> This paragraph has a blue font.
The background color of this page is gray because we changed it with CSS!
</p>
</body></html>
```

Why use external CSS?

a. It keeps your website design and content separate.

b. It is much easier to reuse your CSS code if you have it in a separate file. Instead of typing the same CSS code on every web page you have, simply have many pages refer to a single CSS file with the "link" tag.

c. You can make drastic changes to your web pages with just a few changes in a single CSS file.

2. Internal/embedded CSS

a. This type of CSS is only for single page.

b. When using internal CSS, we must add a new tag, <style>, inside the <head> tag. The HTML code below contains an example of <style>'s usage.

```
<html><head>
<style type="text/css"></style>
</head><body>
<p>Your page's content!</p></body>
</html>
```

Creating internal CSS code

Below is an example of simple CSS code.

```
<html><head>
```

```
<style type="text/css"> p {color: white; }
body {background-color: black; }
</style></head><body>
<p>White text on a black background!</p></body>
</html>
```

3. Inline CSS

    a. It is possible to place CSS right in your HTML code, and this method of CSS usage is referred to as inline css.

    b. Inline CSS has the highest priority out of external, internal, and inline CSS.

    c. This means that you can override styles that are defined in external or internal by using inline CSS.

    d. If you want to add a style inside an HTML element all you have to do is specify the desired CSS properties with the style HTML attribute.

```
<html><head>
<link rel="style sheet" type="text/css" href="test.css" /></head>
<body>
<p style="background: blue; color: white;">A new background
and font color with inline CSS</p></body>
        </html>
```

Explain CSS Background with all its Attributes

CSS background properties are used to define the background effects of an element.

1. CSS background color

    a. The background-color property specifies the background color of an element.

    b. The background color of a page is defined in the body selector:

    c. Below is example of CSS backgrounds

```
body {background-color:#b0c4de;}
```

2. CSS background image

The background-image property specifies an image to use as the background of an element.

```
body {background-image:url('paper.gif');}
```

3. Background image repeat

You can have a background image repeat vertically (y-axis), horizontally (x-axis), in both directions, or in neither direction.

```
p {background-image: url(smallPic.jpg); background-repeat: repeat; }
```

```
h4 {background-image: url(smallPic.jpg); background-repeat: repeat-y; } ol
{background-image: url(smallPic.jpg); background-repeat: repeat-x; }
```

```
ul {background-image: url(smallPic.jpg);background-repeat: no-repeat;}
```

4. CSS fixed background image

The background-attachment property sets whether a background image is fixed or scrolls with the rest of the page.

textarea.noScroll { background-image: url(smallPic.jpg); background-attachment: fixed;} textarea {

background-image: url(smallPic.jpg); background-attachment: scroll;}

5. CSS background image positioning

The background-position property sets the starting position of a background image.

p {background-image: url(smallPic.jpg); background-position: 20px 10px;} h4 {background-image: url(smallPic.jpg); background-position: 30% 30%;}

Explain CSS Lists with all its attributes

The CSS list properties allow you to:

a. Set different list item markers for ordered lists
b. Set different list item markers for unordered lists
c. Set an image as the list item marker

Introduction to CSS3

1. CSS3 is the latest standard for CSS.
2. CSS3 is completely backwards-compatible with earlier versions of CSS.
3. CSS3 has been split into "modules". It contains the "old CSS specification" (which has been split into smaller pieces). In addition, new modules are added.
4. CSS3 Transitions are a presentational effect which allow property changes in CSS values, such as those that may be defined to occur on: hover or: focus, to occur smoothly over a specified duration—rather than happening instantaneously as is the normal behaviour.
5. Transition effects can be applied to a wide variety of CSS properties, including background-color, width, height, opacity, and many more.

Some of the most important CSS3 modules are:

a. Selectors
b. Box model
c. Backgrounds and borders
d. Image values and replaced content
e. Text effects
f. 2D/3D transformations
g. Animations
h. Multiple column layout
i. User interface

What is JavaScript?

1. HTML and CSS concentrate on a static rendering of a page; things do not change on the page over time, or because of events.

2. To do these things, we use scripting languages, which allow content to change dynamically.
3. Not only this, but it is possible to interact with the user beyond what is possible with HTML.
4. Scripts are programs just like any other programming language; they can execute on the client side or the server.

Differentiate between Server Side and Client Side Scripting Languages

Client-side scripting languages

1. The client-side environment used to run scripts is usually a browser.
2. The processing takes place on the end users computer.
3. The source code is transferred from the web server to the user's computer over the internet and run directly in the browser.
4. The scripting language needs to be enabled on the client computer.
5. Sometimes if a user is conscious of security risks they may switch the scripting facility off.
6. When this is the case a message usually pops up to alert the user when script is attempting to run.

Server-side scripting languages

1. The server-side environment that runs a scripting language is a web server.
2. A user's request is fulfilled by running a script directly on the web server to generate dynamic HTML pages.
3. This HTML is then sent to the client browser.
4. It is usually used to provide interactive web sites that interface to databases or other data stores on the server.
5. This is different from client-side scripting where scripts are run by the viewing web browser, usually in JavaScript.
6. The primary advantage to server-side scripting is the ability to highly customize the response based on the user's requirements, access rights, or queries into data stores.

What is Difference between JavaScript and JAVA?

Java is a statically typed language; JavaScript is dynamic

1. Java is class-based; JavaScript is prototype-based.
2. Java constructors are special functions that can only be called at object creation; JavaScript "constructors" are just standard functions.
3. Java requires all non-block statements to end with a semicolon; JavaScript inserts semicolons at the ends of certain lines.
4. Java uses block-based scoping; JavaScript uses function-based scoping.

Java has an implicit this scope for non-static methods, and implicit class scope; JavaScript has implicit global scope.

JavaScript Operators

1. Operators in JavaScript are very similar to operators that appear in other programming languages.

2. The definition of an operator is a symbol that is used to perform an operation.
3. Most often these operations are arithmetic (addition, subtraction, etc.), but not always.

Table 3.10: JavaScript operators

Operator	Name
+	Addition
–	Subtraction
*	Multiplication
/	Division
%	Modulus
=	Assignment

XML

What is XSL?

a. XSL stands for extensible style sheet language.
b. XSL = Style sheets for XML
c. XSL describes how the XML document should be displayed!
d. XSL - More than a style sheet language
e. XSL consists of three parts:
 f. XSLTa language for transforming XML documents
g. XPatha language for navigating in XML documents
h. XSLFOa language for formatting XML documents

What is XSLT?

a. XSLT stands for XSL transformations.
b. XSLT is the most important part of XSL.
c. XSLT transforms an XML document into another XML document.

Explain XSL Transformation and XSL Elements

a. The style sheet provides the template that transforms the document from one structure to another.
b. In this case <xsl:template> starts the definition of the actual template, as the root of the source XML document.
c. The match = "/" attribute makes sure this begins applying the template to the root of the source XML document.

Linking

The style sheet is linked into the XML by adding the connecting statement to the XML document:

```
<?xml-style sheet type="text/xsl" href="libstyle.xsl" ?>
```

XSL Transformations

1. XSLT is the most important part of XSL.
2. XSLT is used to transform an XML document into another XML document, or another type of document that is recognized by a browser, like HTML and

XHTML. Normally XSLT does this by transforming each XML element into an (X)HTML element.

3. With XSLT you can add/remove elements and attributes to or from the output file. You can also rearrange and sort elements, perform tests and make decisions about which elements to hide and display, and a lot more.

4. A common way to describe the transformation process is to say that XSLT transforms an XML source-tree into an XML result-tree.

5. XSLT uses XPath:
   a. XSLT uses XPath to find information in an XML document.
   b. XPath is used to navigate through elements and attributes in XML documents.

6. XSLT works as:
   a. In the transformation process, XSLT uses XPath to define parts of the source document that should match one or more predefined templates.
   b. When a match is found, XSLT will transform the matching part of the source document into the result document.

XSL Elements

XSL contains many elements that can be used to manipulate, iterate and select XML, for output.
   a. Value-of
   b. For-each
   c. Sort
   d. If
   e. Choose

<xsl:value•of> Element

The <xsl:value-of> element extracts the value of a selected node.

The <xsl:value-of> element can be used to select the value of an XML element and add it to the output.

Syntax

<xsl:value-of select="expression" />

expression: This is required. An XPath expression that specifies which node/attribute to extract the value from. It works like navigating a file system where a forward slash (/) selects subdirectories.

<xsl:for•each> Element

The XSL <xsl:for-each> element can be used to select every XML element of a specified node-set.

<xsl:if> Element

To put a conditional if test against the content of the XML file, add an <xsl:if> element to the XSL document.

Syntax

```
<xsl:if test="expression">
...some output if the expression is true...
</xsl:if>
```

\<xsl:sort> Element

The \<xsl:sort> element is used to sort the output.

\<xsl:sort select="artist"/>

The select attribute indicates what XML element to sort on.

\<xsl:choose> Element

The \<xsl:choose> element is used in conjunction with \<xsl:when> and \<xsl:otherwise> to express multiple conditional tests.

Syntax

```
<xsl:choose>
    <xsl:when test="expression">
        ... some output ...
    </xsl:when>
    <xsl:otherwise>
        ... some output ....
    </xsl:otherwise>
</xsl:choose>
```

\<xsl:apply-templates> Element

The \<xsl:apply-templates> element applies a template to the current element or to the current element's child nodes.

If we add a select attribute to the \<xsl:apply-templates> element it will process only the child element that matches the value of the attribute. We can use the select attribute to specify the order in which the child nodes are processed.

Look at the following XSL style sheet:

```
<?xml version="1.0" encoding="ISO-8859-1"?>

<xsl:stylesheet version="1.0"
xmlns:xsl="http://www.w3.org/1999/XSL/Transform">

<xsl:template match="/">
<html>
<body>
<h2>My CD Collection</h2>
<xsl:apply-templates/>
</body>
</html>
</xsl:template>

<xsl:template match="cd">
<p>
<xsl:apply-templates select="title"/>
<xsl:apply-templates select="artist"/>
</p>
```

```
</xsl:template>
</xsl:stylesheet>
```

Introduction to Web Server and Servers

Web servers are computers that deliver (*serves up*) Web pages. Every Web server has an IP address and possibly a domain name. For example, if you enter the URL *http://www.webopedia.com/index.html* in your browser, this sends a request to the Web server whose domain name is *webopedia.com*. The server then fetches the page named *index.html* and sends it to your browser.

Any computer can be turned into a Web server by installing server software and connecting the machine to the Internet. There are many Web server software applications, including public domain software and commercial packages.

Definition—what does Web Server mean?

A web server is a system that delivers content or services to end users over the internet. A web server consists of a physical server, server operating system (OS) and software used to facilitate

HTTP Communication

Web Server

1. A Web Server is computer and the program installed on it. Web Server interacts with the client through the browser. It delivers the web pages to the client and to an application by using the web browser and HTTP protocol respectively.
2. We can also define the web server as the package of larger number of programs installed on a computer connected to internet or intranet for downloading the requested files using File Transfer Protocol, serving e-mail and building and publishing web pages.

Apache web server: Apache Web Server is designed to create web servers that have the ability to host one or more HTTP-based websites. Notable features include the ability to support multiple programming languages, server-side scripting, an authentication mechanism and database support. Apache Web Server can be enhanced by manipulating the code base or adding multiple extensions/add-ons.

It is also widely used by web hosting companies for the purpose of providing shared/virtual hosting, as by default, Apache Web Server supports and distinguishes between different hosts that reside on the same machine.

We have the Following Web Servers

1. Apache1.1
2. WAMP
3. XAMPP

1. Apache web server

a. The Apache web Server, commonly referred to as Apache is web server software notable for playing a key role in the initial growth of the World Wide Web.
b. The first version of Apache, based on the NCSA httpd Web server, was developed in 1995.

c. Apache server has been developed by an open source community—Apache Software Foundation, whose members are constantly adding new useful functionalities

d. The original version of Apache was written for UNIX, but there are now versions that run under OS/2, Windows and other platforms.

e. The Apache Server provides full range of Web Server features, including CGI, SSL and virtual domains. Apache also supports plug-in modules for extensibility.

f. It was called Apache because it was developed from existing NCSA code plus various patches, hence the name a patchy server, or Apache server.

g. Apache is open source free software distributed by the Apache Software Foundation.

h. Apache is reliable, free and relatively easy to configure.

2. WAMP

WAMP is an acronym for Windows, Apache, MySQL and PHP. It is a combination of independently created software's bundled together into a SINGLE installation package to set up a SERVER on your machine with out any hassles. It comes with the GPL License. Contents Of WAMP Server (Package)

3. XAMPP

XAMPP is a small and light Apache distribution containing the most common web development technologies in a single package. Its contents, small size, and portability make it the ideal tool for students developing and testing applications in PHP and MySQL

IIS web server: Stands for "Internet Information Services." IIS is a web server software package designed for Windows Server. It is used for hosting websites and other content on the Web.

Microsoft's Internet Information Services provides a graphical user interface (GUI) for managing websites and the associated users. It provides a visual means of creating, configuring, and publishing sites on the web. The IIS Manager tool allows web administrators to modify website options, such as default pages, error pages, logging settings, security settings, and performance optimizations.

IIS can serve both standard HTML webpages and dynamic webpages, such as ASP. NET applications and PHP pages. When a visitor accesses a page on a static website, IIS simply sends the HTML and associated images to the user's browser. When a page on a dynamic website is accessed, IIS runs any applications and processes any scripts contained in the page, then sends the resulting data to the user's browser.

While IIS includes all the features necessary to host a website, it also supports extensions (or "modules") that add extra functionality to the server. For example, the WinCache Extension enables PHP scripts to run faster by caching PHP processes. The URL Rewrite module allows webmasters to publish pages with friendly URLs that are easier for visitors to type and remember. A streaming extension can be installed to provide streaming media to website visitors.

IIS is a popular option for commercial websites, since it offers many advanced features and is supported by Microsoft. However, it also requires a commercial license and the pricing increases depending on the number of users. Therefore, Apache

HTTP Server, which is open source and free for unlimited users, remains the most popular web server software.

Databases

A database is a collection of information that's related. Access allows you to manage your information in one database file. Within Access there are four major areas: Tables, Queries, Forms and Reports

1. Tables store your data in your database
2. Queries ask questions about information stored in your tables
3. Forms allow you to view data stored in your tables
4. Reports allow you to print data based on queries/tables that you have created.

My SQL

SQL the language of the relational database

SQL stands for the structured query language

SQL is the standardized language used to access the database

ANSI/SQL defines the SQL standard.

SQL contains three parts

1. **Data definition language** includes statements that help you define the database and its objects, e.g. tables, views, triggers, stored procedures, etc.

2. **Data manipulation language** contains statements that allow you to update and query data.

3. **Data control language** allows you to grant the permissions to a user to access specific data in the database.

MySQL? What?

MySQL's co-founder, monty widenius.

1. The name of MySQL is the combination of My and SQL, MySQL.

2. MySQL is a database management system that allows you to manage relational databases. It is open source software backed by Oracle. It means you can use MySQL without paying a dime. Also, if you want, you can change its source code to suit your needs.

3. Even though MySQL is open source software, you can buy a commercial license version from Oracle to get premium support services.

4. MySQL is pretty easy to master in comparison with other database software like Oracle Database, or Microsoft SQL Server.

5. MySQL can run on various platforms UNIX, Linux, Windows, etc. You can install it on a server or even in a desktop. Besides, MySQL is reliable, scalable, and fast.

6. The official way to pronounce MySQL is *My Ess Que Ell, not My Sequel*. However, you can pronounce it whatever you like, who cares?

7. If you develop websites or web applications, MySQL is a good choice. MySQL is an essential component of the LAMP stack, which includes Linux, Apache, MySQL, and PHP.

MS Access

Microsoft Access is an information management tool that helps you store information for reference, reporting, and analysis. Microsoft Access helps you analyze large amounts of information, and manage related data more efficiently than Microsoft Excel or other spreadsheet applications. What is My SQL Pharmacy Drug databases are sites where information about drugs and medications are stored, and one of the largest (and most commonly used) drug databases is compiled by the Food and Drug Administration (FDA). The FDA is a federal agency that oversees and controls all medications in the US, which includes:

1. Over-the-counter (OTC) medications
2. Prescription medications
3. Dietary supplements
4. Vaccines

The FDA drug database includes most of the drugs they have approved in the US since 1939. Best of all, this database is extremely easy to use. To search this database, you simply need to go to the FDA drug databases website. Once you get to this website, you are able to search the database by typing in the name of the drug or by typing in any active ingredient of a drug.

Additionally, the FDA drug database can be used to search drugs that are currently going through clinical trials and/or the approval process. The FDA must approve a drug before it is legally able to be sold and used in the US. Therefore, drug companies must formally submit an application to the FDA for the drug to be approved. The drugs that have not been submitted to the FDA but not yet approved can be found in this database.

ISOLATED KEY POINTS

1. **Browsers:** Browsers are the interpreters of the web. They request information and then when they receive it, they show us on the page in a format we can see and understand.

   Google chrome—currently, the most popular browser brought to you by Google

   Safari—Apple's web browser

   Firefox—open-source browser supported by the Mozilla Foundation

   Internet explorer—Microsoft's browser. You will most often hear web developers complain about this one.

2. **HTML:** HTML is a markup language. It provides the structure of a website so that web browsers know what to show.

3. **CSS:** CSS is a cascading style sheet. CSS let's web designers change colors, fonts, animations, and transitions on the web. They make the web look good.

   LESS—a CSS pre-compiler to make working with CSS easier and add functionality

   SASS—a CSS pre-compiler to make working with CSS easier and add functionality

4. **Programming languages:** Programming languages are ways to communicate to computers and tell them what to do. There are many different programming languages just like there are many different lingual languages (English, Spanish, French, Chinese, etc). One is not better than the other. Developers typically are just

proficient at a couple so they promote those more than others. Below are just some of the languages and links to their homepages.

JavaScript—used by all web browsers, Meteor, and lots of other frameworks

C offeescript—is a kind of "dialect" of JavaScript. It is viewed as simpler and easier on your eyes as a developer but it complies (converts) back into JavaScript

Python—used by the Django framework and used in a lot of mathematical calculations

Ruby—used by the Ruby on Rails framework

PHP—used by Wordpress

Go—newer language, built for speed.

Objective-C—the programming language behind iOS (your iPhone), lead by Apple

Swift—Apple's newest programming language

Java—used by Android (Google) and a lot of desktop applications.

5. **Frameworks:** Frameworks are built to make building and working with programming languages easier. Frameworks typically take all the difficult, repetitive tasks in setting up a new web application and either does them for you or make them very easy for you to do.

Bootstrap—a UI (user interface) framework for building with HTML/CSS/JavaScript

Foundation—a UI framework for building with HTML/CSS/JavaScript

Wordpress—a CMS (content management system) built on PHP. Currently, about 20% of all websites run on this framework

Drupal—a CMS framework built using PHP

NET—a full-stack framework built by Microsoft

Angular.js—a front-end JavaScript framework

Ember.js—a front-end JavaScript framework

Backbone.js—a front-end JavaScript framework.

6. **Libraries:** Libraries are groupings of code snippets to enable a large amount of functionality without having to write it all by yourself. Libraries typically also go through the trouble to make sure the code is efficient and works well across browsers and devices (not always the case, but typically they do).

7. **Databases:** Databases are where all your data is stored. It is like a bunch of filing cabinets with folders filled with files. Databases come mainly in two flavors: SQL and NoSQL. SQL provides more structure which helps with making sure all the data is correct and validated. NoSQL provides a lot of flexibility for building and maintaining applications.

MySQL—It is another popular open-sourced SQL database. MySQL is used in Wordpress websites.

Oracle—It is an enterprise SQL database.

SQL server—It is an SQL server manager created by Microsoft.

8. **Client (or Client-side):** A client is one user of an application. It is you and me when we visit http://google.com. Client's can be desktop computers, tablets, or mobile devices. There are typically multiple clients interacting with the same application stored on a server.

9. **Server (or Server-side):** A server is where the application code is typically stored. Requests are made to the server from clients, and the server will gather the appropriate information and respond to those requests.

10. **Front-end:** The front-end is comprised of HTML, CSS, and JavaScript. This is how and where the website is shown to users.

11. **Back-end:** The back-end is comprised of your server and database. It is the place where functions, methods, and data manipulation happens that you do not want the clients to see.

12. **Protocols:** Protocols are standardized instructions for how to pass information back and forth between computers and devices.

    HTTP—this protocol is how each website gets to your browser. Whenever you type a website like "http://google.com" this protocol requests the website from google's server and then receives a response with the HTML, CSS, and JavaScript of the website.

13. **API:** An API is an application programming interface. It is created by the developer of an application to allow other developers to use some of the application's functionality without sharing code. Developers expose "end points" which are like inputs and outputs of the application. Using an API can control access with API keys. Examples of good API's are those created by Facebook, Twitter, and Google for their web services.

14. **Data formats:** Data formats are the structure of how data is stored.

    JSON—It is quickly becoming the most popular data format

    XML—It was the main data format early in the web days and predominantly used by Microsoft systems

    CSV—It is data formatted by commas. Excel data is typically formatted this way.

PRACTICE QUESTIONS

Long Questions

1. What are Tags in HTML?
2. How to create a hyperlink in HTML?
3. What are the features of XML?
4. What are the differences between HTML and XML?
5. What are the different variations of CSS?
6. What are the CSS frameworks?
7. Write a method which will remove any given character from a String?
8. What is database? What is SQL?

9. What are the different types of database?

10. Explain to the web based server?

OBJECTIVE TYPE QUESTIONS

1. Which is the first Internet search engine?
   a. Google
   b. Archie
   c. Altavista
   d. WAIS

2. In a JavaScript Application what function can be used to send messages to users requesting for an text input?
   a. Display()
   b. Alert()
   c. GetOutput()
   d. Prompt()

3. Assume that an HTML form is designed to purchase the furniture. All the items required are being checked. After selecting the items the payment details are entered and the submit button is pressed. From the following options which one would you prefer to send the data to the server. Assume that all the security is handled.
   a. Only POST
   b. Only GET
   c. Either of GET or POST
   d. Neither GET nor POST

4. Which of the following statements are true?
   a. HTTP runs over TCP
   b. HTTP allows information to be stored in a URL
   c. HTTP can be used to test the validity of a hypertext link
   d. All of the above

5. Which of the following objects can be used in expression and scriplets in JSP without explicitly declaring them?
   a. Request and response only
   b. Response and session only
   c. Session and request only
   d. Session, request and response

6. Which of the following is an Open Source DBMS?
   a. MySQL
   b. Microsoft SQL server
   c. Microsoft access
   d. Oracle

ANSWERS KEY

1. **Archie**
   Explanation: No explanation is available for this question!

2. **Prompt()**
   Explanation: This function is used when we want to input text in JavaScript.

3. **Either of GET or POST**

   Explanation: For sending the data to the server either of them can be used.

4. **All of the above**

   Explanation: No explanation is required for this question!

5. **Session and request only**

   Explanation: Implicit objects in JSP are session: The session object for the client. **Request:** The request triggering the execution of the JSP page.

6. **MySQL**

   Explanation: No explanation is required for this question!

Application of Computers in Pharmacy

COMPUTER

A computer is a programmable machine designed to perform sequence of operations to generate the desired output. It takes data as input, processes the data and produces the output. Earlier the computer was originally defined as a super fast calculator. It had the capacity to solve complex arithmetic and scientific problems at very high speed. But nowadays in addition to handling complex arithmetic computations, computers perform many other tasks like accepting, sorting, selecting, moving, comparing various types of information.

Why Computers are Required in Pharmacy

"The Science of collection, evaluation, organization and dissemination of information by computers" has innumerable applications in the field of healthcare.

Properties

1. Large storage capacity
2. Speed and accuracy
3. Flexibility
4. Repetitive tools
5. Multiple user capacity
6. Ease of transmission

Drug Information Storage and Retrieval

Availability of authentic drug information is the key to promote rational use of drugs, a well accepted concept in clinical practice in the developed world. Drug information is an essential element in achieving health goals and information is an aid to decision making. The objectives of drug information center is to collect information, to evaluate and compare drugs, to provide an education and teaching aid for healthcare personnel, to assist clinicians in the selection of safe and effective medication and to enable pharmacists and pharmacy students to develop their abilities in providing information on drugs and medicines.

Information retrieval (IR) is the activity of obtaining information from large collections of information sources in response to a need.

The working of information retrieval process is explained below:

1. The process of information retrieval starts when a user creates any query into the system through some graphical interface provided.
2. These user-defined queries are the statements of needed information, e.g. queries fork by users in search engines.
3. In IR single query does not match to the right data object instead it matches with the several collections of data objects from which the most relevant document is taken into consideration for further evaluation.
4. The ranking of relevant documents is done to find out the most related document to the given query.
5. This is the key difference between the database searching and information retrieval.
6. After the query is sent to the core of the system. This part has the access to the content management module which is directly linked with the back-end, i.e. the large collections of data objects.
7. Once results R are generated by the core system then it is returned to the user by some graphical user interfaces.
8. The process repeats and results are modified until the user satisfied for what he is actually looking for.

The storage, retrieval, and dissemination of information constitute a major function of any drug information service (DIS). We developed a computerized system for the storage and retrieval of data from drug information requests (DIR) using a MUMPS-based information system. In the past, DIR forms were stored in loose-leaf binders and filed chronologically. Due to the success and increased use of our DIS, this manual filing system became inadequate and awkward to use. Our solution was to develop a computer system where data could be entered from DIR forms and retrieved rapidly and easily. Each DIR was reviewed and key data elements were selected for input. The DIS files may now be searched online rapidly and efficiently. The MUMPS-based information system has provided open access for all staff pharmacists, 24 hours a day. The benefits have been an increase in both the quantity and quality of drug information provided.

Here, we will create a Drug Information Storage and Retrieval System Using MS Access. Before that Let have a sight on Introduction to MS Access.

Introduction

A database is an organized collection of data, generally stored and accessed electronically from a computer system. Where databases are more complex they are often developed using formal design and modeling techniques.

Database objects are the main players in an Access database. Altogether, we have six different types of database objects. From these we'll use Table to create database and Queries to retrieve the stored drug information.

Tables store information. Tables are the heart of any database, and you can create as many tables as you need to store different types of information. A drug databases of marketed drugs contain trade name, dosage form, and strength, they usually do not allocate a unit of prescription or route of administration to the trade name. Apart this, electronic dose calculation, the relation between the denominator of strength and prescribed unit also available software in coded form. When you want to review, add, change, or delete data from the database, consider using a query. Using a query, you can answer very specific questions about the data that would be difficult to answer by looking at table data directly. You can use queries to filter your data, to perform calculations with your data, and to summarize your data. You can also use queries to automate many data management tasks and to review changes in your data before you commit to those changes.

Creating a Table

Create a table with by using the suitable fields and data type respectively.

Creating Queries

1. On the **Create** tab, click **Query Design**.
2. In the **Show Table** dialog box, on the **Tables** tab, double-click Products/Tables you created.
3. Close the **Show Table** dialog box.
4. In the products table, double-click **Fields** to add these fields to the query design grid below (design grid: The grid that you use to design a query or filter in query Design view or in the Advanced Filter/Sort window. For queries, this grid was formerly known as the QBE grid.).
5. Add criteria to field the you want to be asked on Query RUN, to show filtered record according to the query entered (Fig. 4.1).

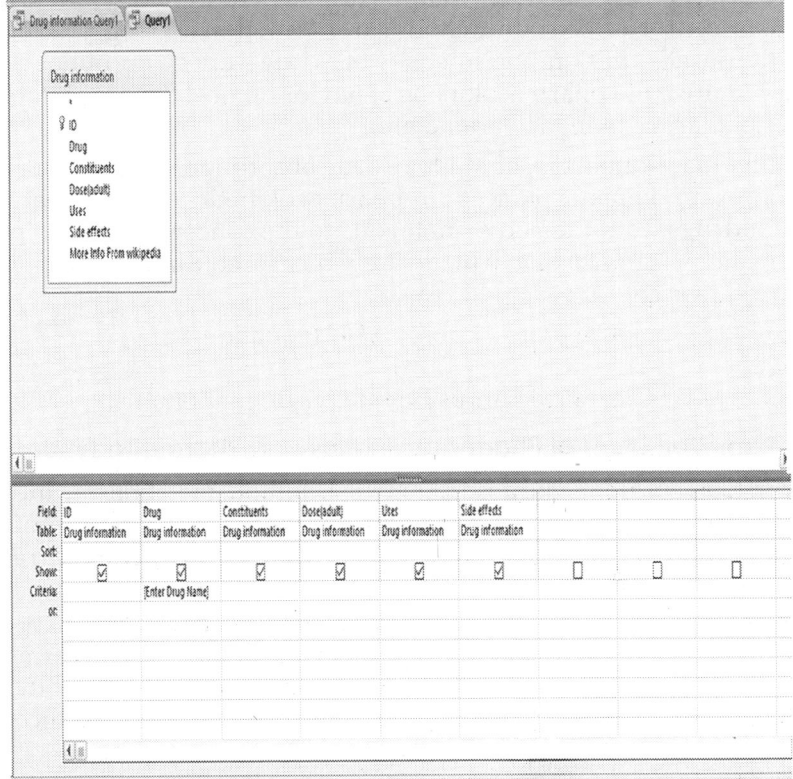

Fig. 4.1: Creating queries

6. On the **Design** tab, in the **Results** group, click **Run**. Enter the Field Value and click OK.

The query runs, and then displays a list of Fields and their records. This is called retrieval of records.

Pharmacokinetics

Pharmacokinetics, sometimes described as what the body does to a drug, refers to the movement of drug into, through, and out of the body—the time course of its absorption, bioavailability, distribution, metabolism, and excretion.

Pharmacokinetics of a drug depends on patient-related factors as well as on the drug's chemical properties. Some patient-related factors (e.g. renal function, genetic makeup, sex, age) can be used to predict the pharmacokinetic parameters in populations. For example, the half-life of some drugs, especially those that require both metabolism and excretion, may be remarkably long in the elderly. Other factors are related to individual physiology. The effects of some individual factors (e.g. renal failure, obesity, hepatic failure, dehydration) can be reasonably predicted, but other factors are idiosyncratic and thus have unpredictable effects. Because of individual differences, drug administration must be based on each patient's needs—traditionally, by empirically adjusting dosage until the therapeutic objective is met. This approach is frequently inadequate because it can delay optimal response or result in adverse effects.

Pharmacodynamics: Described as what a drug does to the body, involves receptor binding, postreceptor effects, and chemical interactions. Drug pharmacokinetics determines the onset, duration, and intensity of a drug's effect. Formulas relating these processes summarize the pharmacokinetic behavior of most drugs (*see* table Formulas Defining Basic Pharmacokinetic Parameters).

Definition: Pharmacokinetics is the study of drug absorption, distribution, metabolism, and excretion. A fundamental concept in pharmacokinetics is drug clearance, that is, elimination of drugs from the body, analogous to the concept of creatinine clearance. In clinical practice, clearance of a drug is rarely measured directly but is calculated as either of the following:

$$Clearance = dose/AUC \text{ (equation 1)}$$
$$or$$
$$Clearance = infusion\ rate/C_{ss} \text{ (equation 2)}$$

Schematic Representation of Pharmacokinetics and Pharmacodynamics

Pharmacokinetics represents the absorption, distribution, metabolism, and elimination of drugs from the body. **Pharmacodynamics** describes the interaction of drugs with target tissues. GI = gastrointestinal; IM = intramuscular; IP = intraperitoneal; IV = intravenous; PO = by mouth; SC = subcutaneous.

AUC, the area under the curve, represents the total drug exposure integrated over time and is an important parameter for both pharmacokinetic and pharmacodynamic analyses. As indicated in equation 1, the clearance is simply the ratio of the dose to the AUC, so that the higher the AUC for a given dose, the lower the clearance. If a drug is administered by continuous infusion and a steady state is achieved, the clearance can be estimated from a single measurement of the plasma drug concentration (C_{ss}) as in equation 2.

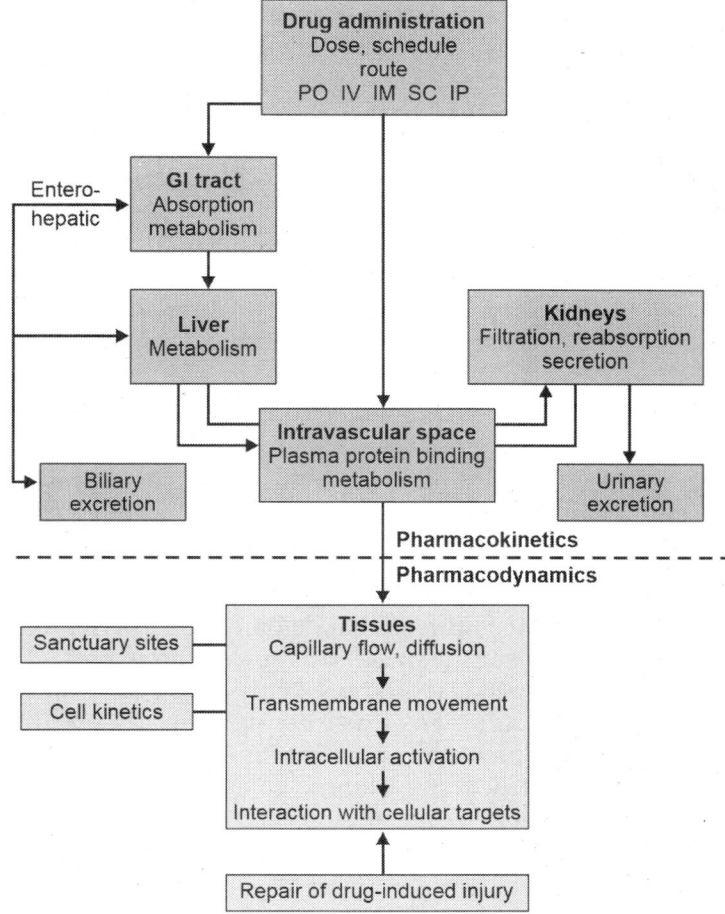

Fig. 4.2: Schematic representation of pharmacokinetics and pharmacodynamics

Clearance can conceptually be considered to be a function of both distribution and elimination. In the simplest pharmacokinetic model,

$$\text{Clearance} = VK \text{ (equation 3)}$$

V is the volume of distribution, and K is the elimination constant. V is the volume of fluid in which the dose is initially diluted, and thus the higher the V, the lower the initial concentration. K is the elimination constant, which is inversely proportional to the half-life, the period of time that must elapse to reach a 50% decrease in plasma concentration. When the half-life is short, K is high and plasma concentrations decline rapidly. Thus both a high V and a high K result in relatively low plasma concentrations and a high clearance.

Linear Pharmacokinetic Models

Although pharmacokinetic analysis can be conducted without specifying any mathematical models (non-compartmental methods), it is helpful to use such models as guides in therapeutic decision-making. There are several important characteristics of drugs that have linear pharmacokinetics. The key feature of a linear pharmacokinetic model is that.

This indicates that the instantaneous rate of change in drug concentration depends only on the current concentration. The half-life will remain constant, no matter how high the concentration.

One implication of this principle is that the drug exposure (AUC) is not affected by changes in drug schedule. For example, the AUC after a 60 mg/m² bolus dose of doxorubicin equals the total AUC for 3 daily (or weekly) bolus doses of 20 mg/m², which equals the AUC for the same dose administered as a 96-hour infusion. A second implication is that the AUC is proportional to the dose. Thus, if one measures the AUC for a 60 mg/m² dose, one can estimate the AUC for a 90 mg/m² dose in the same patient as being 50% greater.

The simplest linear pharmacokinetic model, shown graphically is shown below:

$$C(t) = \frac{Dose}{V}(e^{-kt}) \text{ (equation 5)}$$

After the infusion is terminated, the drug concentration decays at the same rate as if it had been administered as an instantaneous bolus. Thus, if T represents the infusion time, then the postinfusion drug concentrations can be represented as

$$C(t) = C\,(T)e^{-k(t-T)} \text{ (equation 7)}$$

A large variety of computer software is available for pharmacokinetic analysis. The interested reader is likely to benefit from hands on experience with such programs. Several caveats need to be emphasized for the casual reader. The validity of pharmacokinetic modeling depends to a large extent on the quality of the data entered into the model. Thus, drug infusions must be precisely timed, plasma samples must be obtained on schedule, and analytical methods must be sensitive and specific. The data must be properly weighted to avoid bias due to the increased probability of analytical errors at drug concentrations near the detection limit of the assay. Results obtained using a specific model should be compared to those using non-compartmental methods.

Non-Linear Pharmacokinetic Models

Non-linear pharmacokinetic models imply that some aspect of the pharmacokinetic behavior of the drug is saturable. The mathematics of non-linear models are beyond the scope of this chapter, but the principles are very relevant to several anticancer agents. In contrast to the administration schedule of drugs with linear pharmacokinetics, alteration of the administration schedule of drugs that display non-linear kinetics may markedly affect the AUC and potentially alter clinical effects.

Non-linear pharmacokinetic behavior commonly occurs when there is saturation of a major metabolic pathway. This results in decreased clearance at higher doses, with a greater than proportional increase in the AUC. The AUC will also increase if the infusion duration is shortened, due to slower clearance at the higher peak plasma concentrations. This is clearly the case for 5-FU, probably due to saturation of its conversion to dihydrofluorouracil by the enzyme dihydropyrimidine dehydrogenase. Schaaf and colleagues demonstrated that doubling of the 5-FU dose from approximately 7.5 to 15 mg/kg (by IV bolus) resulted in a 135% increase in the mean AUC. Since 5-FU is used on a variety of schedules, its non-linear pharmacokinetic behavior may be one factor in its highly schedule-dependent effects. Paclitaxel has also been demonstrated to have nonlinear pharmacokinetics. Thus, the AUC is higher, for a fixed dose.

MATHEMATICAL MODEL IN DRUG DESIGN
Introduction

During the last decade the pharmaceutical industry has followed a simplistic assumption that a single drug hitting a single target was the \"rational" way to design drugs. That was a direct consequence of our lack of knowledge about function-determining features of desired ligand molecules in the drug discovery process.

Mathematical Model in Drug Design can be Divided in Three Parts
1. Drug or Poison?

During the life a human body absorbs different substances, which have to be metabolized. For instance, for a toxic ligand a docking to a certain protein in the body can prevent a intoxication of the organism. Thus, the development of fast and accurate protein ligand docking simulations is of high interest and helps to understand in advance whether a substance is toxic or not.

2. Bone Growth

The remodelling of bone depends on the interaction and concentration of osteoclasts, osteoblasts and additional substances (i.e. osteocysts). This interaction is controlled by hormones. The mathematical modelling and the simulation of the hormones with focus on their influence on bone remodelling is considered.

3. Markov Operator Projection

In computational drug design the binding process of small molecules to their target proteins is important. The binding process can be described by transition rates or also by transition probabilities. However, these two concepts do not directly fit together (they do not commute).

Multiscales in Biomolecules

Bridging the scale from quantum mechanics to molecular dynamics for proteins and drug design.

Hospital and Clinical Pharmacy

Clinical and hospital pharmacy deals with the application of drug treatments to patients in a hospital or clinical setting.

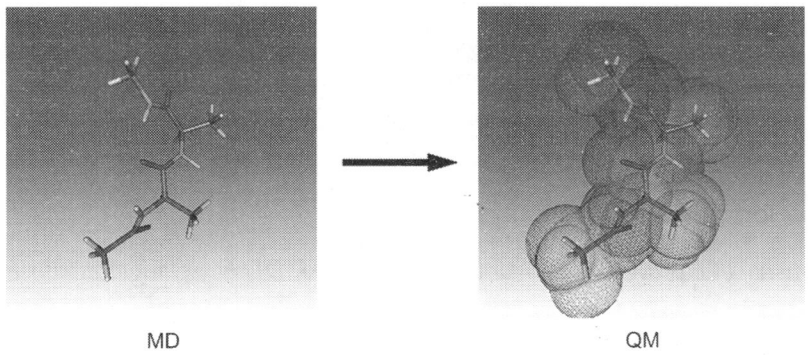

MD   QM

Fig. 4.3: Multiscales in biomolecules

Inside Clinical and Hospital Pharmacy

The study of pharmacy involves the effective recommendation and administration of various medications for the safety and health of patients. Clinical or hospital pharmacy is a specialization of this field that includes additional duties such as aiding doctors in applying drug therapies. Typically, pharmacology students can choose to specialize in this area during their residency program.

Hospital and Clinical Pharmacy personnel can be divided into three major categories:

1. **Management:** Management includes the chief pharmacist and sometimes deputy chief pharmacists, who are responsible for procurement, distribution, and control of all pharmaceuticals used within the institution and for management of personnel within the pharmacy department.
2. **Professional staff:** These professionals are qualified pharmacists who procure, distribute, and control medications and supervise support staff for these activities. In some facilities, pharmacists provide clinical consulting services and medicine information.
3. **Support staff:** The support staff category often includes a combination of trained pharmacy technicians, clerical personnel, and messengers.

The smallest hospitals may have only two or three pharmacy staff members, with the chief pharmacist as the only pharmacist. Larger teaching hospitals that provide extensive pharmaceutical distribution and clinical services may have more than 100 staff members.

The cornerstone for a well-functioning medication system is an up-to-date manual of policies and procedures. Staff members should be familiar with the manual and adhere to it.

Physical Organization

The extent of the pharmacy's physical facility is determined by the size of the hospital and the services provided. A large pharmacy department might have the following sections within one physical space or in separate locations throughout the hospital:

1. Administrative offices
2. Bulk storage
3. Narcotic or dangerous drug locker
4. Manufacturing and repackaging
5. Intravenous solution compounding
6. Inpatient and outpatient dispensing
7. Medicine information resource center
8. After-hours pharmacy
9. Emergency medicine storage

Multiple-department Pharmacy System

Source: Ministry of Health, Government of Kenya, 1994. DDA = Dangerous Drugs Act.

Note: Forms and registers for wards, operating room, special areas, and outpatient department (OPD) injection room are the same as for the central pharmacy system.

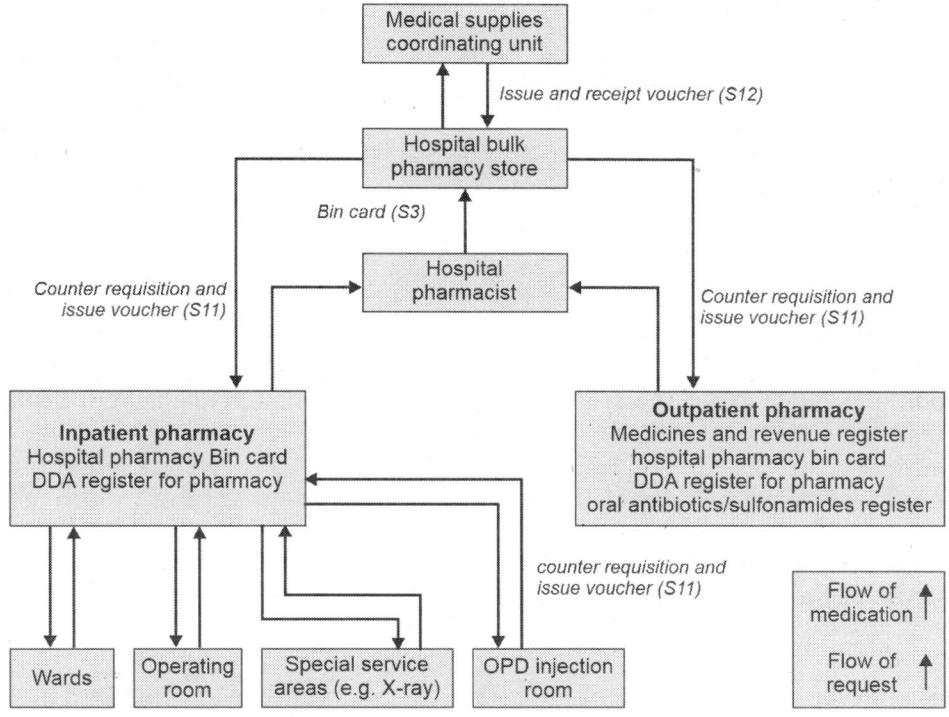

Fig. 4.4: Multiple-department pharmacy system

Electronic Prescribing and Discharge

E-prescribing, or electronic prescribing is a technology framework that allows physicians and other medical practitioners to write and send prescriptions to a participating pharmacy electronically instead of using handwritten or faxed notes or calling in prescriptions.

Electronic prescribing (e-prescribing or **e-Rx)** is the computer-based electronic generation, transmission, and filling of a medical prescription, taking the place of paper and faxed prescriptions. E-prescribing allows a physician, pharmacist, nurse practitioner, or physician assistant to use digital prescription software to electronically transmit a new prescription or renewal authorization to a community or mail-order pharmacy. It outlines the ability to send error-free, accurate, and understandable prescriptions electronically from the healthcare provider to the pharmacy. E-prescribing is meant to reduce the risks associated with traditional prescription script writing. It is also one of the major reasons for the push for electronic medical records. By sharing medical prescription information, e-prescribing seeks to connect the patient's team of healthcare providers to facilitate knowledgeable decision-making.

Introduction

Electronic prescribing was introduced into EGP practices in the early 1990s in an attempt to improve accuracy and efficiency and should now be fully operational. Similar progress has not been made in hospital practice.

The Connecting for Health (previously National Programme for Information Technology) e-prescribing programme aims to improve patient safety by facilitating the development and delivery of electronic prescribing systems. Connecting for Health recently stated that implementation will be challenging and will require acceptance of new ways of working.

Working with the National Patient Safety Agency, Connecting for Health published guidelines recently on design-related safety features to be incorporated into electronic systems. This follows studies in hospitals in the UK where electronic prescribing systems are in place. Nationally, there is a range of systems, not all of which are compatible with each other.

Bar Code Medicine Identification and Automated Dispensing of Drugs

Bar code technology in healthcare is the use of optical machine-readable representation of data in a hospital or healthcare setting.

The American Society of Health-System Pharmacists encourages hospital and health-system pharmacies to incorporate bar code scanning into inventory management, dose preparation and packaging, and dispensing of medications. The purpose of such scanning is to ensure that drug products distributed, deployed to intermediate storage areas, or used in the preparation of patient doses are the correct products, are in date, and have not been recalled. Such bar code scanning should be employed in:

1. Stocking of inventory both in the pharmacy and in other locations from which patient medications may be dispensed (e.g. an automated dispensing device).
2. Manual packaging of oral solid and liquid medications.
3. Compounding, repackaging, and labeling processes (e.g. scanning of source ingredients).
4. Retrieving medications from automated dispensing devices.
5. Dispensing from the pharmacy to any location. Prudent use of bar coding technology in these processes will enhance patient safety and the quality of care by improving the accuracy of core pharmacy functions, closing potential gaps in the bar code-assisted medication administration (BCMA) process, and allowing better allocation of pharmacists' knowledge and skills.

Benefits of Bar Code Verification During Inventory, Preparation, and Dispensing

Initial estimates of the contribution of pharmacy dispensing errors to the overall medication errors were quite low. However, recent reports have suggested that adding bar coding to the pharmacy dispensing process can significantly reduce opportunities for medication errors at the bedside and reduce the occurrence of potential adverse drug reactions. Incorporating bar code scanning in inventory management, dose preparation and packaging, and dispensing can improve patient safety in the following ways:

1. Scanning during stocking in the pharmacy or patient-care locations (e.g. loading of an automated dispensing device) can help ensure that the product is placed in the correct location.
2. Scanning during the retrieval of medications mitigates the hazards of erroneous medication stocking, which is especially important in the case of automated dispensing devices, where there is a potential risk that caregivers will override controls and remove medications for immediate use.

3. Scanning of source ingredients during compounding, repackaging, or labeling processes can ensure that labeled doses contain the appropriate ingredients. Additionally, such scanning creates a reliable link be the entire system, as the system cannot properly recognize and evaluate the drug products being scanned. Procedures should address such issues as the expected behavior while scanning occurs, specific prohibited acts, and the penalties associated with known at-risk behavior.

Mobile Technology and Adherence Monitoring

Mobile technology provides opportunities for pharmacists and other healthcare providers to help improve and assess patients' medication adherence.

The topic of using technology to improve medication adherence is not new, as many innovators and companies have tried over the years to create products that patients would use in their daily lives. Inevitably, most patients stick with the tried-and-true pill box because it works.

How Mobile Technology is Impacting Pharmacy?

Mobile technology has an ever-increasing role in driving efficiency, accuracy, and improved financial performance in pharmacies of every type and size.

Monitoring Drug Adherence

Nonadherence to medical recommendations is a leading cause of morbidity and mortality in a wide array of disease processes in all age groups. Adherence is especially important in patients with chronic or complex medical conditions such as transplantation, who need to adhere to lifelong medication and dietary regimens. For these individuals, adherence is of the utmost importance given its association with health outcomes.

Extensive data strongly suggests that nonadherence is a significant cause of morbidity and mortality in post-transplant patients. More specifically, nonadherence to immunosuppressant therapy is considered to be the leading cause of preventable graft failure, contributing to 20% of late acute rejection episodes and 16% of graft losses within the overall transplant population. Yet, in clinical practice, there lacks a systematic approach to identifying and treating nonadherence.

Measurement of Adherence

There is no gold standard for the measurement of adherence, and each proposed method has its shortcomings. A comprehensive review of assessment methods is beyond the scope of this manuscript; however, a brief summary and analysis is warranted. Methods of measuring nonadherence fall into two different groups:

1. Direct measures of adherence including observed therapy and measurement of drug/metabolite levels.
2. Indirect measures including patient surveys, rate of prescription refills, electronic medication monitoring, and medical record documentation. Each method has its limitations, and many techniques remain to be validated.

An "ideal" measure of nonadherence should be objective, direct, pose little burden to the patient, and provide actionable information about patient adherence to the clinical team (and perhaps even to the patient herself/himself and other caretakers).

Unfortunately, in the clinical setting, most measurements of nonadherence include subjective methods such as self-report via questionnaires or clinician-documented observations in an electronic medical record (EMR).

Diagnostic Systems

Diagnostic systems is a global leader of products and instruments used for diagnosing infectious diseases. Our products are used in the clinical market to screen for microbial presence, grow and identify organisms, and test for antibiotic susceptibility.

It is a natural phenomenon that is also shaped by society and culture. It is biological but also behavioral and social. Mental illness is a problem of both the brain and the mind, and this ambiguity presents a challenge for those who seek to accurately classify psychiatric disorders.

The terms "diagnostics" and "diagnoses" have been around for a very long time, though our understanding of them has changed. The first and oldest wave of diagnostics involved easily measurable values, such as age, weight, gender, skin color, and eye color. While these diagnostics are simple in nature, their value should not be underscored; indeed, some of them remain better prognostic indicators than more technologically advanced diagnostics. The second wave of diagnostics arrived with the implementation of novel tools and newer technologies. Significant advances in the understanding of basic human biology, health, and disease were provided by the abilities to measure more subtle and individualistic physical signs and symptoms, as well as the technologies to evaluate bacterial cultures and gather and interpret biological biopsies. The third wave of diagnostics is a fairly recent phenomenon, and new, interesting discoveries have led to as much confusion as they have clarity. As the scope of diagnostics has grown, so have the duties and responsibilities of those involved. Historically, this tended not to directly involve pharmacists, but that is rapidly changing.

Diagnostic-linked treatment decisions are increasing at a staggering pace. Although empirical treatments in which a practitioner may not know a patient's specific issues are becoming the exception instead of the rule, diagnostics remains uncharted territory for pharmacists in all practice settings. Like the proverbial train on the tracks, it is approaching quickly whether we like it or not, and our lack of awareness of this area will not protect us from being run over.

Lab-diagnostic System

Diagnostic Systems Laboratories is a leading source of specialized immunodiagnostic products for clinical, research, academic and veterinary markets worldwide. DSL currently offers more than 200 immunoassays and over 430 research reagents for growth factors, fertility and reproduction, androgen assessment, bone and mineral metabolism, thyroid function, energy homeostasis and obesity testing.

Point-of-care testing (POCT) is traditionally defined as laboratory diagnostics performed at or near the site where clinical care is delivered. POCT thereby combines sample collection, analysis, and reporting of results into a robust integrated testing structure, with a simple user interface. The availability of reliable devices and consolidated tests for patient screening, diagnosis and monitoring has allowed broad diffusion of POCT to the patient's bedside, physician offices, pharmacies, other healthcare facilities, supermarkets, and even into the patient's home. However, current evidence clearly shows that POCT can be subjective, and might even amplify the traditional problems encountered in the preanalytical, analytical and postanalytical phases of the total testing process. This may especially be seen in inappropriateness of the test request, collection of unsuitable biological materials, inaccurate test performances, larger analytical imprecision, unsuitable report formatting, delayed reporting of critical value, and report recording/retrieval. POCT patient care service in the pharmacy can be regarded as a valuable option for the present and future since it might be beneficial for all parties. However, several economic, clinical and regulatory issues should also be addressed before this opportunity can turn into a real advantage for patients and the entire healthcare system. The most appropriate allocation of POCT within the diagnostic pathway, as well as its adjuvant role in screening, diagnosis and monitoring of diseases should also be clearly established in order to prevent widespread and deregulated implementation.

Patient Monitoring System

What Is Patient Monitoring?

Continuous measurement of patient parameters, such as heart rate and rhythm, respiratory rate, blood pressure, blood-oxygen saturation, and many other parameters have become a common feature of the care of critically ill patients. When accurate and immediate decision-making is crucial for effective patient care, electronic monitors frequently are used to collect and display physiological data. Increasingly, such data are collected using noninvasive sensors from less seriously ill patients in a hospital's medical-surgical units, labor and delivery suites, nursing homes, or patients' own homes to detect unexpected life-threatening conditions or to record routine but required data efficiently. **Patient monitoring** can be rigorously defined as "repeated or continuous observations or measurements of the patient, his or her physiological function, and the function of life support equipment, for the purpose of guiding management decisions, including when to make therapeutic interventions, and assessment of those interventions".

Patient Monitoring in Intensive Care Units

There are at least five categories of patients who need physiological monitoring:

1. Patients with unstable physiological regulatory systems, e.g. a patient whose respiratory system is suppressed by a drug overdose or anesthesia
2. Patients with a suspected life-threatening condition, e.g. a patient who has findings indicating an acute myocardial infarction (heart attack)
3. Patients at high-risk of developing a life-threatening condition, e.g. patients immediately after open-heart surgery or a premature infant whose heart and lungs are not fully developed
4. Patients in a critical physiological state, e.g. patients with multiple trauma or septic shock.
5. Mother and baby during the labor and delivery process.

 A nurse at a patient's ICU bedside. Above the nurse's head is the bedside monitor which measurse and displays key physiological data, above her left hand is an IV pump connected to a Medical Information Bus (MIB), to her right are two screens of a patient ventilator and to the far right is a bedside computer terminal used for data entry and data review. (*Source:* Courtesy of Dr Reed M Gardner).

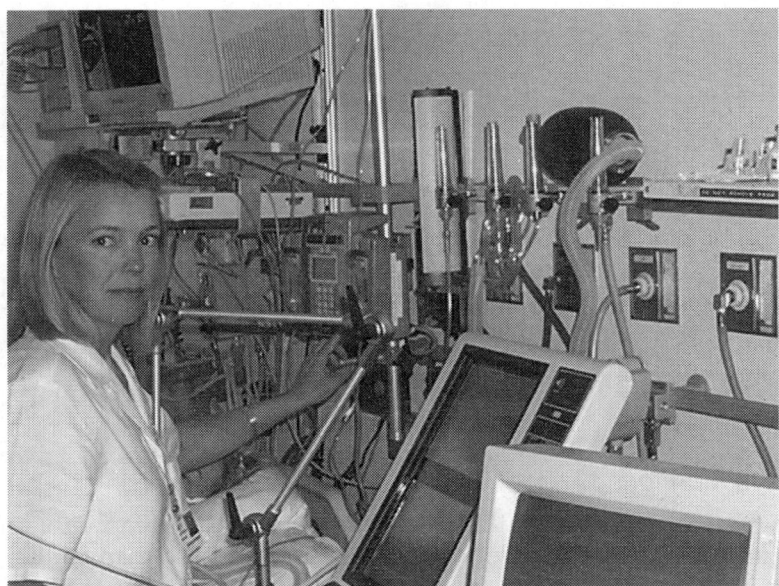

Fig. 4.5: Patient monitoring in intensive care units

Pharmacy Information System

A **pharmacy information system (PIS)** is a system that has many different functions in order to maintain the supply and organization of drugs. It can be a separate system for pharmacy usage only, or it can be coordinated with an inpatient hospital computer physician order entry (CPOE) system. A PIS paired with a CPOE allows for an easier transfer of information.

A PIS is used to reduce medication errors, increase patient safety, report drug usage, and track costs. Inpatient pharmacy information systems are used in the hospital setting while outpatient pharmacy information systems are used in home settings for discharged patients, clinics, long-term care facilities, and home healthcare. Most of the uses and capabilities of the PIS are similar for inpatient and outpatient settings. However, the outpatient PIS has a stronger emphasis on medication labeling, drug warnings, and instructions for administration.

Pharmacy Information System Necessities

Josh tells Julie that a PIS has many different uses that are helpful for multiple departments in a medical organization. He explains each necessary part of the PIS and the ways in which the pharmacist uses it.

1. **A user interface** is beneficial to all departments and allows the pharmacist to organize and select the orders to place in a patient profile, work on multiple orders at one time, and show detailed patient profiles.

2. **Security** is also important. With so many departments having some type of access to the connected computer system, only certain departments need access to certain parts of the system.

3. **A data retention** plan is also helpful in a PIS so that records are kept for a year or longer to help pharmacists and physicians understand the cost and usage of

drugs. Pharmacists can use patient records to keep track of clinical screenings, what medications they are on, and what recommendations they may need regarding healthcare.

ISOLATED KEY POINTS

- Computers in pharmacy are used for the information of drug data, records and files, drug management (creating, modifying, adding and deleting data in patient files to generate reports), business details.
- Applications of computers in pharmacy
  - i. Providing a receipt for the patient
  - ii. Record of transaction of money
  - iii. Ordering low quantity of products via electronic transitions
  - iv. Generation of multiple analysis for day, week, month for number of prescription handles and amounts of cash
  - v. Estimation of profits and financial rational analysis
  - vi. Printing of billing and payment details
  - vii. Inventory control purpose
  - viii. Whenever the drugs or medicaments are added to the stock or else removed from stock; the position of stock gets updated instantaneously
  - ix. Records of various drug data, i.e. drug data information
  - x. Computers are useful for getting the complete drug information which is used to satisfy the queries by patients about toxicology, adverse drug reactions, and drug-drug and drug-food interactions.
  - xi. Drug Bank Data Base gives complete and detailed description of drug (pharmacological and pharmaceutical action) and also involves bioinformatics and cheminformation.

PRACTICE QUESTIONS

Long Answer Type Questions

1. The computer is assisting the human being in almost every activity. Explain?
2. Explain drug information storage and retrieval in detail?
3. Explain the applications of computer in hospital pharmacy?
4. Explain the tools for hospital pharmacy process improvement?
5. Benefits and limitations of computerization?

OBJECTIVE TYPE QUESTIONS

1. A word processor can be used to:
   - a. Write text
   - b. Edit text
   - c. Print text
   - d. All of these

2. **Use of computer in education is started in:**
   a. 1960s
   b. 1970s
   c. 1980s
   d. 1990s

3. **Sesame oil belongs to family:**
   a. Graminae
   b. Ephorbiaceae
   c. Leguminosae
   d. Pedialiaceae

4. **The leaves of Tylophora indica are used in the treatment of:**
   a. Asthma
   b. General debility
   c. Cough
   d. Itch

5. **The solution used to rinse vagina is called:**
   a. Douches
   b. Irrigation
   c. Enema
   d. Diluent

ANSWERS KEY

1. d   2. b   3. a   4. a   5. b

Bioinformatics in Computers

BIOINFORMATICS

Bioinformatics is an interdisciplinary field that develops methods and software tools for understanding biological data. As an interdisciplinary field of science, bioinformatics combines biology, computer science, information engineering, mathematics and statistics to analyze and interpret biological data. Bioinformatics includes biological studies that use computer programming as part of their methodology, as well as a specific analysis "pipelines" that are repeatedly used, particularly in the field of genomics.

Introduction

Bioinformatics involves the integration of computers, software tools, and databases in an effort to address biological questions. Bioinformatics approaches are often used for major initiatives that generate large data sets. Two important large-scale activities that use bioinformatics are genomics and proteomics.

Genomics refers to the analysis of genomes. A genome can be thought of as the complete set of DNA sequences that codes for the hereditary material that is passed on from generation to generation. Thus, genomics refers to the sequencing and analysis of all of these genomic entities, including genes and transcripts, in an organism.

Proteomics, on the other hand, refers to the analysis of the complete set of proteins or proteome. In addition to genomics and proteomics, there are many more areas of biology where bioinformatics is being applied (i.e. metabolomics, transcriptomics). Each of these important areas in bioinformatics aims to understand complex biological systems (Fig. 5.1).

The Wheel of Biological Understanding. System biology strives to understand all aspects of an organism and its environment through the combination of a variety of scientific fields.

Bioinformatics can be applied from single cells to whole ecosystems. By understanding the complete "parts lists" in a genome, scientists are gaining a better understanding of complex biological systems. Understanding the interactions that occur between all of these parts in a genome or proteome represents the next level of complexity in the system. Through these approaches, bioinformatics has the potential to offer key insights into our understanding and modeling of how specific human diseases or healthy states manifest themselves.

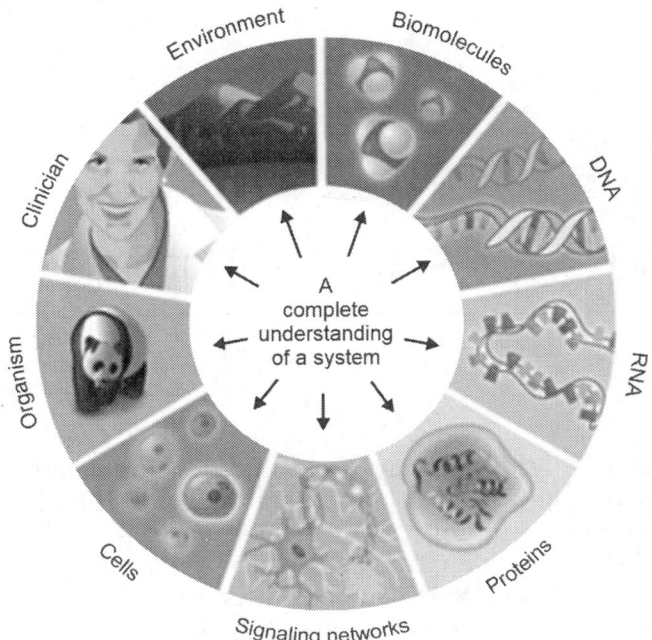

Fig. 5.1: Bioinformatics

Bioinformatics has become an important part of many areas of biology. In experimental molecular biology, bioinformatics techniques such as image and signal processing allow extraction of useful results from large amounts of raw data. In the field of genetics, it aids in sequencing and annotating genomes and their observed mutations. It plays a role in the analysis of gene and protein expression and regulation. In structural biology, it aids in the simulation and modeling of DNA, RNA, proteins as well as biomolecular interactions.

Objectives of Bioinformatics

The field of bioinformatics has three main objectives:

1. To organize vast reams of molecular biology data in an efficient manner.
2. To develop tools that aid in the analysis of such data.
3. To interpret the results accurately and meaningfully.

The advent and rapid rise of bioinformatics has been due to the massive increases in computing power and laboratory technology in recent years. These advances have made it possible to process and analyze the digital information—DNA, genes and genomes—at the heart of life itself.

As bioinformatics can be used in any system where information can be represented digitally, it can be applied across the entire spectrum of living organisms, from single cells to complex ecosystems.

To get an idea of the staggering amounts of data and information that bioinformatics has to deal with, consider the human genome. A genome is an organism's complete set of DNA. DNA molecules are made of two twisting, paired strands, and each strand is made of nucleotide bases Adenine (A), Thymine (T), Guanine (G), and Cytosine (C). The human genome contains about 3 billion of these base pairs. Genome sequencing involved figuring out the exact order of all 3 billion of these DNA nucleotides, a feat which would not have been possible without massive amounts of computing power.

Bioinformatics Databases

"A biological database is a large, organized body of persistent data, usually associated with computerized software designed to update, query, and retrieve components of the data stored within the system. A simple database might be a single file containing many records, each of which includes the same set of information."

A few popular databases are GenBank from NCBI (National Center for Biotechnology Information), SwissProt from the Swiss Institute of Bioinformatics and PIR from the Protein Information Resource.

GenBank: GenBank (Genetic Sequence Databank) is one of the fastest growing repositories of known genetic sequences.

EMBL: The EMBL Nucleotide Sequence Database is a comprehensive database of DNA and RNA sequences collected from the scientific literature and patent applications and directly submitted from researchers and sequencing groups.

SwissProt: This is a protein sequence database that provides a high level of integration with other databases and also has a very low level of redundancy (means less identical sequences are present in the database).

Kinds of Biological Databases

1. Swiss-Prot and PIR for protein sequences.
2. GenBank and DDBJ for genome sequences.
3. Protein Databank for protein structures (Fig. 5.2).

Application of Bioinformatics

In bioinformatics there are lot of different databases, each focusing on a different aspect of the field from a unique perspective, e.g. organisms, genes, proteins, and diseases. Associations exist between the different databases' data, such as links between genes and proteins, or gene homologs between species. Multiple standardization efforts have resulted in large data warehouses, each of which seeks to be the definitive portal for a particular bioinformatics subcommunity. Each such warehouse provides three services to its community:

1. A data representation, in the form of a schema and query interface with terminology matched to the community.

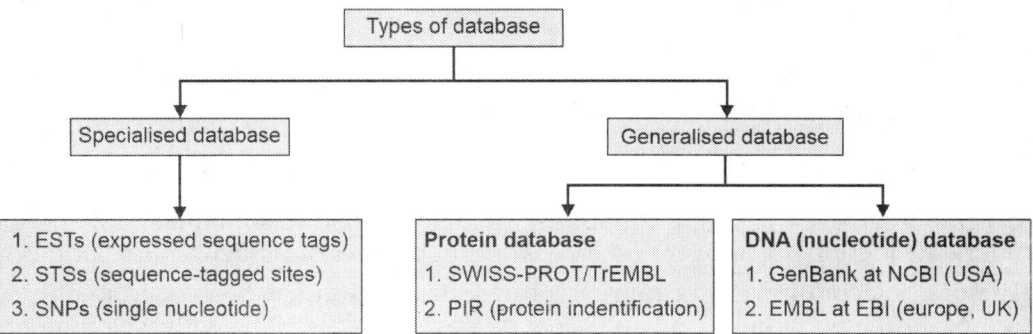

Fig. 5.2: Types of database

2. Access to data, in the form of both raw measurements and statistically or heuristically derived diagnoses and links, e.g. a gene that appears to be correlated with a disease.
3. Cleaning and curation of data produced locally, as well as data that have possibly been imported from elsewhere.

Impact of Bioinformatics in Vaccine Discovery

Due to increase in the concentration of pathogens in the environment, the demands for vaccines to eradicate them at the initial stage are very high. Several methodologies have been tried to diminish the occasions and cost of vaccines, essentially concentrating on the determination of suitable antigens or antigenic structures, bearers, and adjuvant.

One of these methodologies is the inclusion of bioinformatics techniques and investigations into vaccine preparation process.

The following approaches of bioinformatics have been used in vaccine development:

1. Reverse vaccinology
2. Immunoinformatics
3. Structural vaccinology

Vaccines are the pharmaceutical products that offer the best cost benefit ratio in the prevention or treatment of diseases. In that it is a pharmaceutical product, a vaccine development and production are costly and it takes years for this to be accomplished. Several approaches have been applied to reduce the times and costs of their development, mainly focusing on the selection of appropriate antigens or antigenic structures, carriers, and adjuvants. One of these approaches is the incorporation of bioinformatics methods and analyses into vaccine development. At present, there are many alternative strategies to design and develop effective and safe new generation vaccines, based on bioinformatics approaches through reverse vaccinology, immunoinformatics, and structural vaccinology.

Reverse vaccinology, immunoinformatics, and structural vaccinology are described and addressed in the design and development of specific vaccines against infectious diseases caused by bacteria, viruses, and parasites. These include some emerging or reemerging infectious diseases, as well as therapeutic vaccines to fight cancer, allergies, and substance abuse, which have been facilitated and improved by using bioinformatics tools or which are under development based on bioinformatics strategies.

Reverse vaccinology: It is a methodology that uses bioinformatics tools for the identification of structures from bacteria, virus, parasites, cancer cells, or allergens that could induce an immune response capable of protecting against a specific disease.

Immunoinformatics: The immunological system can be classified as cellular or humoral. If a vaccine that induces a cellular response, vaccine is identified by antigens in which histocompatibility complex (MHC) molecules is present in T lymphocytes, e.g. a tuberculosis vaccine or a parasite vaccine against leishmaniasis, while for humoral by identifying antigens for B cells, e.g. in the case of influenza virus or HIV.

Structural vaccinology: This approach to vaccine design has been used mainly to select or design peptide-based vaccines or cross-reactive antigens with the capability of generating immunity against different antigenically divergent pathogens.

ISOLATED KEY POINTS

- Bioinformatics is an interdisciplinary field that develops methods and software tools for understanding biological data.
- Bioinformatics combines biology, computer science, mathematics and statistics to analyze and interpret biological data.
- Bioinformatics involves the integration of computers, software tools, and databases in an effort to address biological questions.
- Two important large-scale activities that use bioinformatics are genomics and proteomics. Genomics refers to the analysis of genomes. A genome can be thought of as the complete set of DNA sequences that codes for the hereditary material that is passed on from generation to generation.
- Proteomics refers to the analysis of the complete set of proteins or proteome.
- Bioinformatics has become an important part of many areas of biology like in experimental molecular biology, bioinformatics techniques such as image and signal processing allow extraction of useful results from large amounts of raw data. In the field of genetics, it aids in sequencing and annotating genomes and their observed mutations.
- Purpose of bioinformatic is to involve the integration of computers, software tools, and databases in an effort to address biological questions.
- Objectives of bioinformatics are:
  - i. To organize vast reams of molecular biology data in an efficient manner.
  - ii. To develop tools that aid in the analysis of such data.
  - iii. To interpret the results accurately and meaningfully.
- To get an idea of the staggering amounts of data and information bioinformatics has to deal with the human genome. A genome is an organism's complete set of DNA.
- DNA molecules are made of two twisting, paired strands, and each strand is made of nucleotide bases Adenine (A), Thymine (T), Guanine (G), and Cytosine (C).
- Bioinformatics database is a large, organized body of persistent data, usually associated with computerized software designed to update, query, and retrieve components of the data stored within the system, e.g. Gen Bank, SwissProt
- Kinds of biological databases are:
  - i. Swiss-Prot and PIR for protein sequences.
  - ii. GenBank and DDBJ for genome sequences.
  - iii. Protein databank for protein structures
- The following approaches of bioinformatics have been used in vaccine development:
  - i. Reverse vaccinology
  - ii. Immunoinformatics
  - iii. Structural vaccinology
- Vaccines are the pharmaceutical products that offer the best cost benefit ratio in the prevention or treatment of diseases.

PRACTICE QUESTIONS

Long Answer Type Questions

1. What is bioinformatics?
2. Which types of issues or problems related to biological data are dealt with the bioinformatics?
3. Which are the main sub-disciplines of bioinformatics?
4. What is medical-informatics?
5. Why do we move towards the use of bioinformatics?
6. Which type of skills are required to be a good bioinformatician?

OBJECTIVE TYPE QUESTIONS

1. Laboratory work using computers and associated web based analysis generally online is referred as:
   a. Dry lab
   b. Web lab
   c. Wet lab
   d. Insilico

2. Step wise method for solving problems in computer science is called:
   a. Flowchart
   b. Sequential design
   c. Procedure
   d. Algorithm

3. The term bioinformatics was coined by:
   a. JD Watson
   b. Margaret Dayhoff
   c. Pauline Hogeweg
   d. Frederic Sanger

4. Phylogenetic relationship can be shown by:
   a. Dendrogram
   b. Gene bank
   c. Data retrieving tool
   d. Data search tool

5. BLOSUM matrices are used for:
   a. Multiple sequence alignment
   b. Pair wise sequence alignment
   c. Phylogenetic analysis
   d. All of the above

6. Which of the following is a nucleotide sequence data base?
   a. EMBL
   b. Swiss prot
   c. Prosite
   d. Trembl

ANSWERS KEY

| 1. b | 2. d | 3. c | 4. a | 5. b | 6. a |

Computer as Data Analysis in Preclinical Development

INTRODUCTION

Computers in preclinical development have become an integral part of pharmaceutical research and development. Computers have found their importance as data management and data analysis tools in Pharmaceutical R and D.

Preclinical development involves the testing of a prospective drug on animals to determine its safety and dose that can be used in humans. After this initial study on animals, an Investigation New Drug (IND) application needs to be filed with the regulatory authorities. An IND application may require as much as 50,000 pages of supporting documentation. The data for every single data point has to be collected, managed, analyzed, reported, audited and finally archived as per the prevailing regulatory laws.

The use of computers has led to efficiently completing the above steps for the data collected hence increasing efficiency and productivity of development. The three computer based systems used to manage majority of the data in the preclinical development stage include the CDS (Chromatographic Data Systems), LIMS (Laboratory Information Management Systems) and TIMS (Text Information Management Systems). There are several vendors available for these each of these systems.

Scientists from many different disciplines participate in pharmaceutical development. Their search areas may be very different, but they all generate scientific data (and text documents), which are the products of development laboratories. Even a typical Investigational New Drug (IND) application requires around 50,000 pages of supporting documents. One way or another, every single data point has to go through the acquiring, analyzing, managing, reporting, auditing, and archiving process according to a set of specific rules and regulations. The wide use of computers has tremendously increased efficiency and productivity in pharmaceutical development.

On the other hand, it has also created unique problems and challenges for the industry. This overview discusses these topics briefly by focusing on the preclinical development area (also known as the area of Chemical Manufacturing and Control, or CMC). Considering the pervasiveness of computer applications in every scientist's daily activities, pecial emphases are put on three widely used computer systems:

  a. CDS

  b. LIMS

  c. TIMS

It may also be beneficial to the reader if we define the sources of the scientific data in preclinical development. Some development activities that generate the majority of the data are:

a. Drug substance/drug product purity, potency, and other testing

b. Drug substance/drug product stability testing

c. Method development, validation, and transfer

d. Drug product formulation development

e. Drug substance/drug product manufacturing process development, validation, and transfer.

Chromatographic Data Systems (CDS)

The importance of CDS is directly related to the roles that chromatography, particularly HPLC and gas chromatography (GC), play in pharmaceutical analysis. HPLC and GC are the main workhorses in pharmaceutical analysis. HPLC, GC and CDS are used for several instrumental analysis technologies.

On compared with the traditional analytical methods, the adoption of chromatographic methods represented a significant improvement in pharmaceutical analysis. This was because chromatographic methods had the advantages of method specificity, the ability to separate and detect low-level impurities. Specificity is especially important for methods intended for early phase drug development when the chemical and physical properties of the active pharmaceutical ingredient (API) are not fully understood and the synthetic processes are not fully developed. Therefore the assurance of safety in clinical trials of an API relies heavily on the ability of analytical methods to detect and quantitate unknown impurities that may pose safety concerns. And, slowly, HPLC and GC established their places as the mainstream analytical methods in pharmaceutical analysis.

The more and more importance chromatographic methods, practical needs prompted instrument vendors to come up with more efficient ways for collecting and processing chromatographic data.

Drawbacks of CDS

1. Because the CDS used a dedicated hardware and wiring system, it was relatively expensive to install.

2. Difficult to scale up because more minicomputers would be needed with increases in the number of users.

3. The performance of the system would degrade as the number of users increased.

As instrumental analysis played an increasingly important part in pharmaceutical development, an ever-larger percentage of the data in Good Manufacturing Practice and/or Good Laboratory Practice (GMP/GLP) studies were captured and stored electronically.

With server-based computing, the applications are deployed, managed, supported, and executed on a dedicated application server. Server-based computing uses a multiuser operating system and a method for distributing the presentation of an application's interface to a client device. There are no software components installed on the client PC. The client's PC simply acts as the application server's display. CDS using this model significantly reduced the total cost in implementation and maintenance and significantly increased its compliance with regulatory guidelines.

The Modern CDS

Use of server-based computing is only one of the important features of the modern CDS. The other two important features are the use of embedded data structure and direct instrument control. The earlier generations of CDS used a directory file structure, meaning that the raw data and other files such as the instrument method and data processing method were stored at separate locations. There would either be no connections or only partial connections between these files. The most significant drawback of this type of file management was the potential for methods and raw data to be accidentally overwritten. To prevent this from happening, the raw data and result files must be locked. If in some cases the locked data needed to be reprocessed, the system administrator must unlock the files. The embedded relational database has been widely used for LIMS and is a much better file structure.

Laboratory Information Management Systems (LIMS)

LIMS represent an integral part of the data management systems used in preclinical development. LIMS are needed partly because CDS cannot provide enough data management capability. For example, CDS cannot handle data from nonchromatographic tests. LIMS is for sample management in preclinical development, more specifically in drug substance and drug product stability studies. LIMS are designed to automate a large part of these stability studies including sample tracking, sample distribution, work assignment, results capturing, data processing, data review and approval, report generation, and data archiving, retrieving, and sharing.

LIMS Hardware and Architectures

By the early 1990s, most LIMS started using commercial relational database technology and client/server systems, which operated on UNIX or the new Windows NT platform. The most advanced LIMS utilize server-based architecture to ensure system security and control.

There are four main types of architectural options when implementing LIMS. The LAN (local area network) installation. In this set-up, the LIMS are installed on both the clients and the server. System administration is required at each facility.

The second type is the WAN (wide area network) installation. In this set-up the LIMS take advantage of telecommunication technology to cover a great distance. The set-up can also be used to connect disparate LANs together.

The third type is the so-called "centrally hosted thin client installation". For this set-up, system administration is managed at a corporate center, where the LIMS are hosted and distributed via a WAN or the Internet with a virtual private network (VPN).

The last and also the newest type is the ASP (Application Service Provision provider)—hosted installation. In this set-up, the LIMS are hosted on a centrally managed server form and maintained by third-party specialists.

Different Types of LIMS

Customer-tailored LIMS—the customer purchases a generic product from the vendor. The vendor and customer will work together over a period of time to configure the software to adapt it to meet end user needs. This usually involves extensive programming, which can be performed by the trained end user or dedicated supporting personnel on the customer side. Programming support is usually needed for the entire life of the LIMS to accommodate changes in development projects.

Preconfigured LIMS—this LIMS does not require extensive customer programming. To meet specific needs of end users, the vendors provide a comprehensive suite of configuration tools. These tools allow end users to add new screens, menus, functions, and reports in a rapid and intuitive manner. The tools also allow the LIMS to be more easily integrated with other business applications such as document processing, spreadsheets, and manufacturing systems.

Specialized LIMS—this type of LIMS is based on the fact that certain laboratories have a range of well-defined processes (e.g. stability testing) that are performed according to a specific set of regulations and by using well-established tests. The tests are done according to industry-wide accepted protocols. Specialized LIMS are tailor-made for certain types of laboratories. Therefore the performance can be optimized for clearly defined work process.

LIMS as rented service—the application service provision provider (ASP) is a means of obtaining access to software applications without the need to acquire expensive licenses and hardware or employ high-cost support resources. The application is hosted on a third-party site with system maintenance, back-up, and recovery provided by a third party. Products and services can be rented for a contract period on a fixed cost per user/per month basis.

Text Information Management Systems (TIMS)

When TIMS is used in today's workflow, the scientist can use a report template to facilitate report writing. Some cut-and-paste procedures are still needed to include data and figures. After the draft report is completed, the scientist can send the reviewers an electronic link for the document. The reviewers can review the document and make changes and corrections with the "tracking change" function. When the review is completed, the author can choose to accept the changes or deny them. If auditing is needed, the same process can be used. The finalized document is issued within the TIMS by adding an issue date and signatures, if necessary, and converting into an unalterable PDF file. Future changes made after issuance are captured through version control. End users can also access the issued document electronically and remotely. Comparison of the new process vs the old one has demonstrated the advantages of TIMS.

Documentation Requirements in Preclinical Development

Product specification documents and analytical test methods—Drug substances and products for clinical trials are tested based on these documents, and so are the stability samples. A manually controlled system would require the analyst to sign out hard copies of the documents from a central location. If TIMS is implemented, the analyst can obtain the documents from the secured database and then the documents should be destroyed after the test is completed.

Current TIMS Products

TIMS used in preclinical text document management usually is a simplified version of ECM. At the highest enterprise platform level, ECM vendors include Documentum,

FileNet, Interwoven, Stellent, and Vignette. At a lower level, the upper-tier products are provided by Day Software, FatWire, and IBM. For less costly products, there are Ingeniux, PaperThin, RedDot Solutions, and Serena Software. It should also be pointed out that the cost of acquiring and maintaining a fully validated TIMS is much higher than that of a non-GMP/GLP system. Therefore many of the non-GMP/GLP documents in early-phase development are managed with nonvalidated TIMS.

ISOLATED KEY POINTS

- **Computers in Preclinical Development:** Some of the key features are as follows:
    i. Computer systems must be validated to ensure consistency of intended purpose, accuracy and reliability.
    ii. Computer systems must provide time based Audit Trial to record actions for creating, modifying or deleting records.
    iii. Access to computer systems used for research must be limited to authorize personnel only.
    iv. Computer systems should have the capability to be configured specific to each user.
    v. Part 11 is a regulatory requirement which has not been enforced by the FDA however this has impacted the CDS, LIMS and TIMS with respect to their design and security capabilities.
- **Chromatography data systems (CDS):** The CDS is used for automating pharmaceutical analysis, mostly those that pertain to chromatographic data generated from various test like HPLC (high performance liquid chromatography), GC (gas chromatography), IC (ion exchange chromatography), CE (capillary electrophoresis and SFC (super critical fluid chromatography).
- **Laboratory information management systems (LIMS):** The LIMS provides data management capability for all non chromatographic data that cannot be handled by the CDS. Another important function of LIMS is automation of stability studies including sample tracking, distribution, work assignment, result capturing, data processing, review, approval, report generation and data archiving, retrieving and sharing.
- **Text information management systems (TIMS):** The TIMS is not used as widely as the LIMS, however, it helps improve efficiency in managing business-critical text documents. However the process of manually writing, reviewing, auditing and publishing text documents is time consuming which is why the industry is working towards the method of electronic submissions. The truth is that we are still not there, and electronic submissions may still take a while to be a reality.

PRACTICE QUESTIONS

Long Answer Type Questions

1. Explain computers in preclinical development.
2. Explain the procedure of chromatography data systems (CDS) in detail.
3. Differentiate between LIMS and TIMS.

4. Explain various data analysis and management tools.

5. Explain the emergency and evolution of CDS.

OBJECTIVE TYPE QUESTIONS

1. Chromatography is used to separate:

    a. Solution   b. Mixtures

    c. Molecules   d. Atoms

2. Chromatography with solid stationary phase is called:

    a. Circle chromatography   b. Square chromatography

    c. Solid chromatography   d. Adsorption chromatography

3. Pattern on the paper in chromatography is called:

    a. Chroming   b. Chroma

    c. Chromatograph   d. Chromatogram

4. Mobile phase can be:

    a. Gas or liquid   b. Solid or liquid

    c. Only solid   d. Only gas

5. Components which have small value of K have affinity for:

    a. Mobile phase   b. Stationary phase

    c. No phase   d. Solution

ANSWERS KEY

1. b   2. d   3. d   4. a   5. b

Experiments in Computers

Create a HTML web page to show personal information.

REQUIREMENTS
- Text editor
- An internet browser

INTRODUCTION

When you navigate to a web page on the Internet, the browser is doing a lot of work. The browser reads all the necessary files (HTML, CSS, and JavaScript) and interprets those raw resources to paint the complex page you see.

In this article, you'll learn how to create a web page using a text editor on your own computer, then view the web page in your browser. If you're interested in publishing your web page to the World Wide Web (the Internet) for everyone to see, check out this article after you understand the steps below.

STEP 1: OPEN YOUR TEXT EDITOR

The first step is to open your text editor. It is important to use a "raw" text editor, and not a formatted word processor.

Word processors insert characters which make the page look good, but aren't valid HTML. They're great tools for making stylish documents, such as academic papers and flyers, but they also insert characters that aren't valid HTML. Since a web page file must contain valid HTML, a text editor is a better tool than a word processor for building web pages.

STEP 2: WRITE YOUR HTML SKELETON

Now that your text editor is open, you can begin writing your HTML. As you learned in the first lesson of the HTML and CSS course, there are a few things that are always present in a well-formatted HTML file. Here's all of them together again:

```
<!DOCTYPE html>

<html>

    <head>
```

```
    <title>My First Web Page!</title>
  </head>
  <body>
    <h1>Hello World!</h1>
  </body>
</html>
```

You can use this exact skeleton if you like. Just copy and paste it into your text editor. Make sure you include everything!

STEP 3: SAVE YOUR FILE

Your web page is now ready, but currently it only exists inside of your text editor. The next step is to save the file to your computer. If you closed the text editor now without saving, your new web page would be lost! There are a few important things to keep in mind when you save it the file:

1. Use the .html, HTML file extension, i.e. about_me.html
2. Don't use any spaces or special characters in the file name. Use underscores (_) or dashes (–) instead.
3. Decide where in your computer you will save the file, and make sure to remember the location!

USE THE .html—HTML FILE EXTENSION

A **file extension** is the suffix of a file name, and describes the type of the file. The file extension is always the last 3 or 4 characters in a filename, preceded by a period. For example, the HTML file extension is .html, and it tells the browser (and other applications) to interpret the contents of the file as a web page. Note that on older web pages you may see .htm, but this archaic and no longer used.

DON'T USE ANY SPACES OR SPECIAL CHARACTERS IN THE FILE NAME

When choosing a file name, keep it simple. Stick to numbers and letters. Use underscores (_) or dashes (–) instead of spaces. Leave out percent signs, slashes, question marks, exclamation points, commas, and other "special characters". The browser needs to locate the file based on its name, and special characters within the file name can interrupt that process. File names should be kept simple and should follow conventions in order to make navigating to your web page more reliable.

DECIDE WHEREIN YOUR COMPUTER YOU WILL SAVE THE FILE

After choosing a file name, select an appropriate location in your file system to save your web page. It is good practice to create a new folder to house this web page. If you do create a new folder, use the same naming conventions outlined above in order to minimize future headaches. The *most important thing* when selecting the location to save to is to *remember where you saved it*. If you saved it already but you don't remember where, just click File>Save As…, choose a new location to save, and be sure to remember this time.

STEP 4: OPEN YOUR WEB PAGE IN YOUR BROWSER

Now you're ready to view your new page in your browser! First, open up your browser. In the top menu, click File>OpenFile. Navigate to the location you saved your web page. Click on your web page file and then click Open. You should see your web page!

PRACTICAL 2

Creating mailing labels Using Label Wizard, generating label in MS WORD

Creating your Mailing Labels

1. Start Microsoft Word.
2. Click the New Document button.

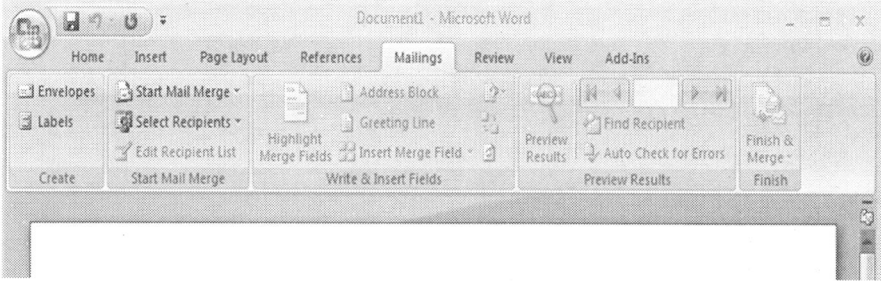

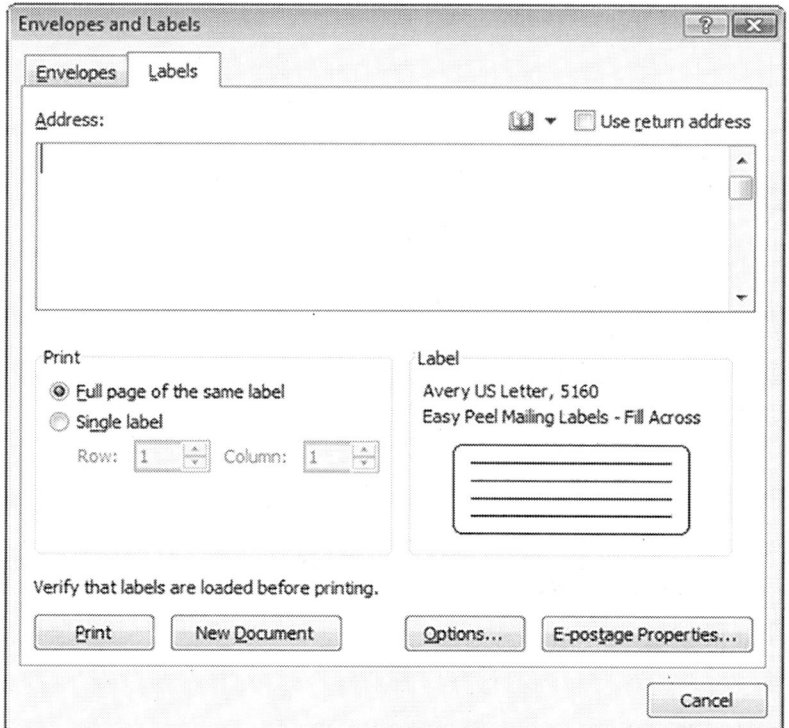

3. From the Tools menu, select Letters and Mailings, then select Envelopes and Labels.
4. Select the Labels tab, click Options, select the type of labels you want to create and then click OK.
5. Click New Document.

Type and Format the Content of your Labels

1. Turn on table gridlines (borders) so that you can see the outline of your labels: from the Table menu, choose Show Gridlines.
2. If you're creating a page of labels that will all look the same, type and format one label, then use copy and paste to create the rest of the labels (see step 5 for details on copy and paste).

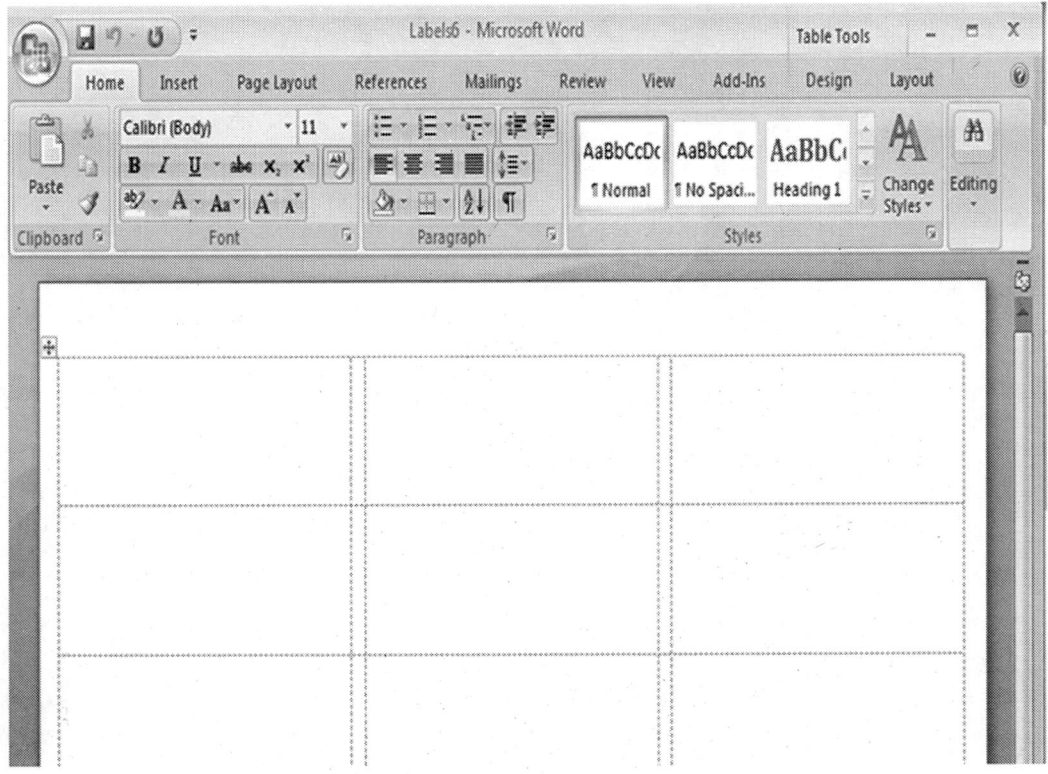

Insert Photos into your Labels

1. Scan your photos.

2. OR

3. Use photos that you have saved on your computer's hard drive.

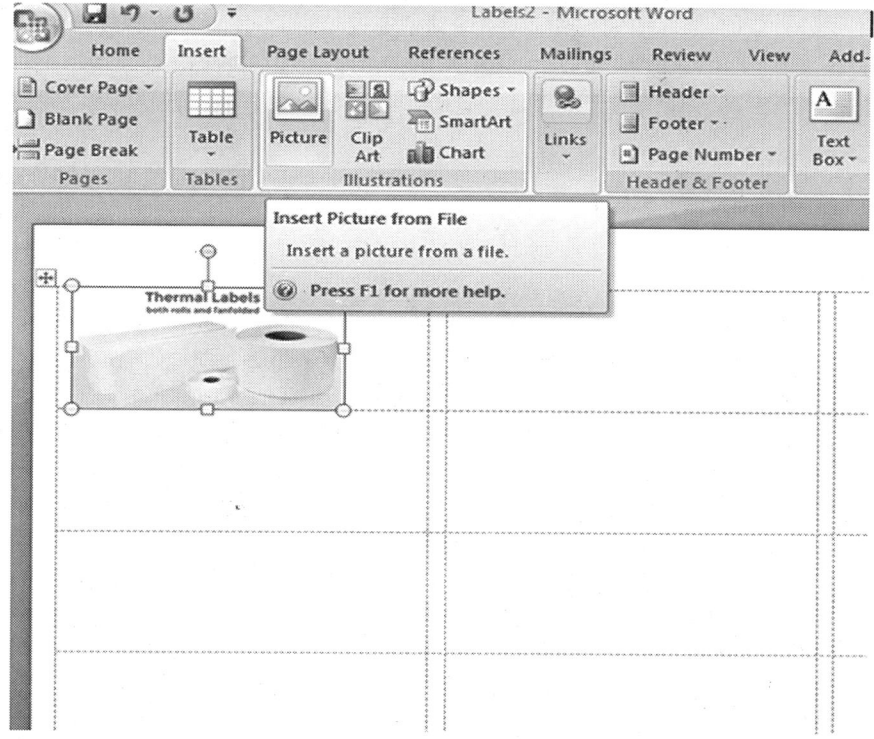

Resize or Move Each Image as Needed so that it Fits in the Label

If you want to duplicate information (text and/or photos) in every label, copy and paste the information into each label.

To do this you need to:

1. Select the text and/or photos you want to duplicate.
2. From the edit menu, select copy
3. Place your cursor in a label where you want to place the information.
4. From the edit menu, select Paste.

Save your Mailing labels

1. From the file menu, select Save.
2. In the save as window, locate and open the folder where you want to save the labels.
3. Type a name for your labels, then click save.

If you want to Preview your Labels

1. From the file menu, select print preview.
2. OR
3. Click the print preview button.
   When you are done previewing, click Close to close the preview window.
   Click on File and press Print.

PRACTICAL 3

Create a database in MS Access to store the patient information with the required fields using access

How to Start Microsoft Access

There are two ways to Start MS Access.

1. From Windows, 'Start' button.
2. From Desktop, Right Click> 'New' option.

Let's have a look of starting MS ACCESS using both the ways:

Option 1: From Windows, Start button.

Step 1: Click on the 'Windows' icon. You will find the list of installed programs.

Step 2: Check and click on Access Icon.

Step 3: MS Access Application window will appear

Steps 4: Press 'Esc'

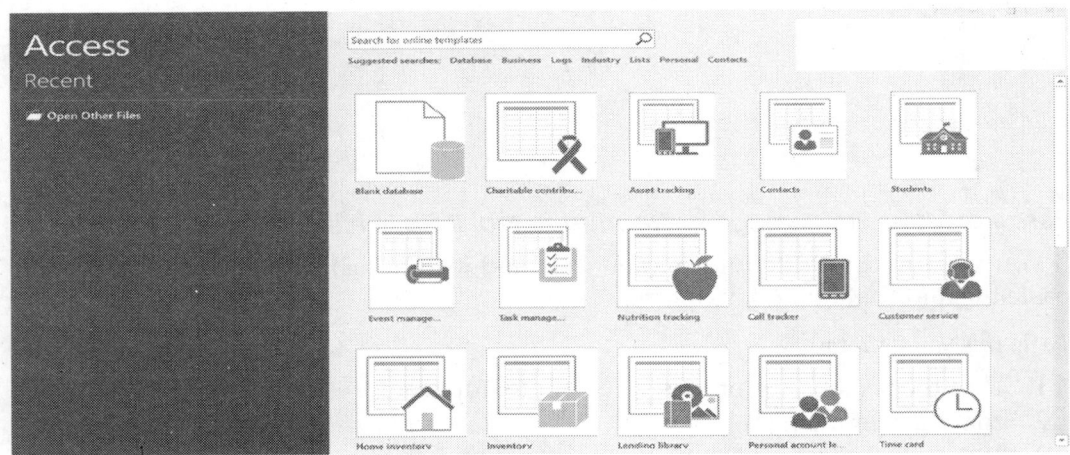

Result: This will open the MS ACCESS windows application

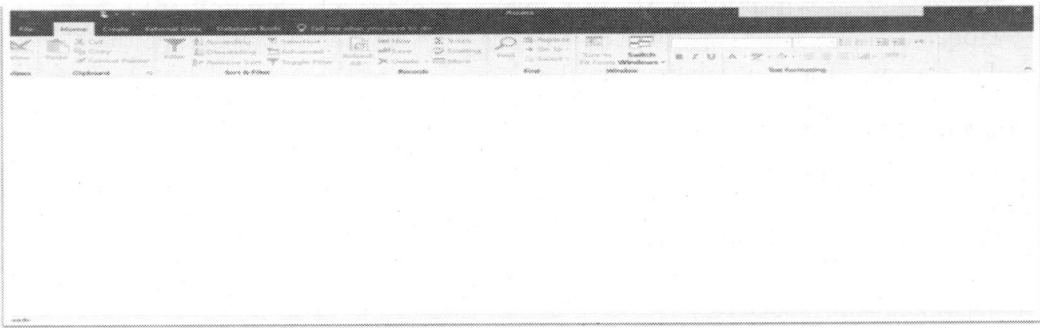

Option 2: From Desktop, 'New' option.

Step 1: Right Click from Desktop and Click 'New'

Step 2: Click on 'Microsoft Access Database Option'

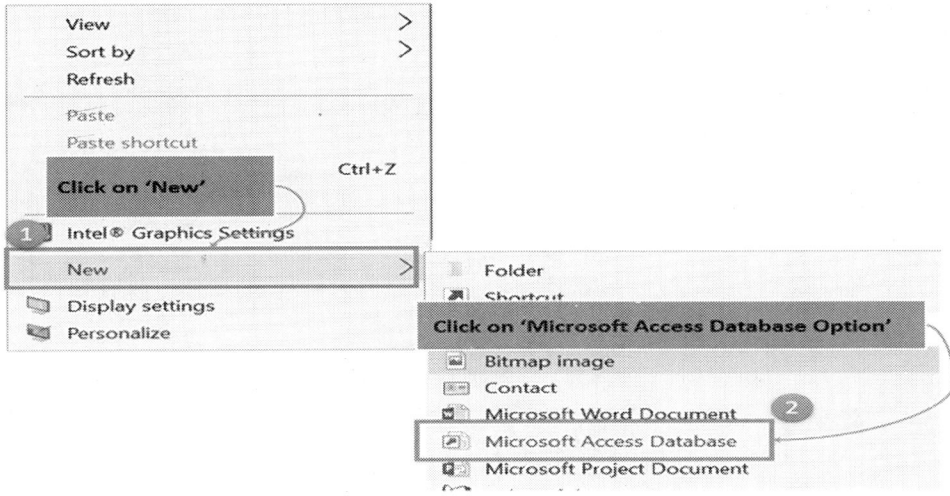

Step 3: MS Access Application window will appear (as shown above)

Step 4: Press 'Esc'

Result: This will open the MS Access windows application (as shown above)

How to Create a Database

Before we create Database, let's quickly understand the holistic picture of what Database is, with particular reference to MS Access.

Let's, start with a few examples in real life:

1. We have Bookcase where Books resides,
2. We have i-pods where we have a collection of music and cases are countless.

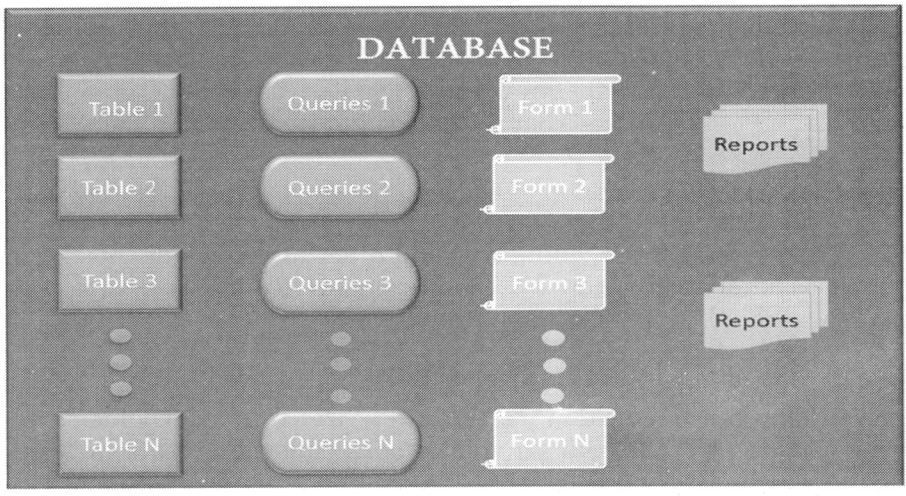

Similarly, we have MS Access Database is a kind of home for all your tables, queries, Forms, Reports, etc. in MS-Access which are interlinked.

Technically, Database store the data in a well-organized manner for easy access and retrieval.

Patient information

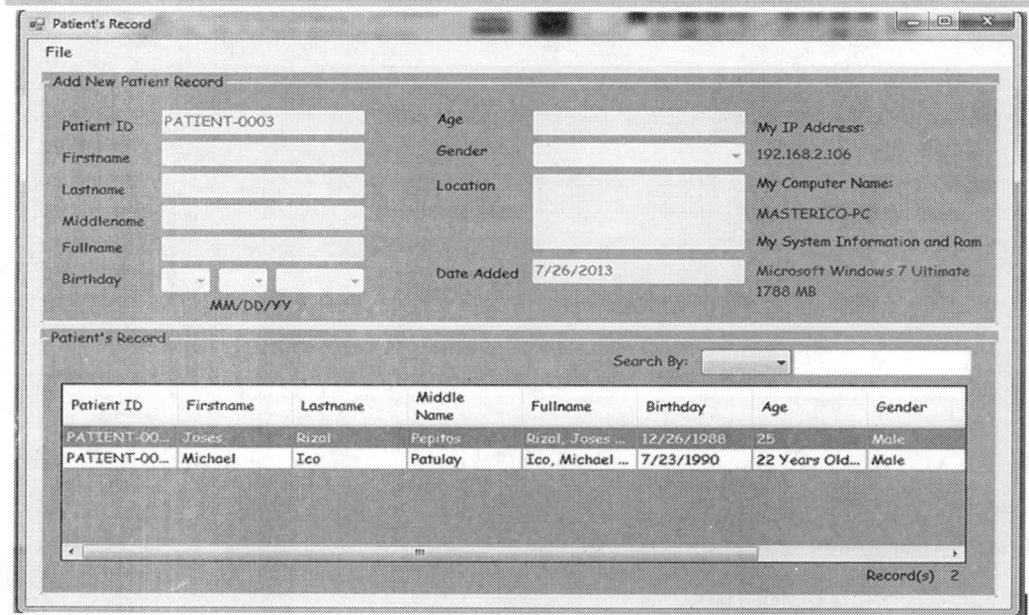

PRACTICAL 4

Creating invoice table using—MS Access

Step 1

Create a "Customer" table that contains all of your customer or client information by clicking the "Table Design" button on the "Create" tab of the ribbon at the top of the page. The "Table Design" tool allows you to create a table from a blank template. Include fields for your customer's name, contact information and unique ID number.

Step 2

Create an "Invoice" table that contains information regarding each business transaction. Add fields for location, cost and other necessary details. To assign a customer to each transaction, add a "Customer Name" field, select "Lookup Wizard" as a data type and link to the "Customer" table.

Step 3

Select the customer's name field in the "Lookup Wizard" to display the names in the "Customer Name" field of your "Invoice" table. This step creates a relationship between the "Customer" and "Invoice" tables, and reduces data redundancy. Instead of typing in the customer's contact information for each business transaction, you store the information just once in the "Customer" table.

Step 4

Create an "Invoice" report by selecting the "Report Wizard" button from the "Create" tab on the ribbon. Select all of your fields in the "Invoice" table and customer contact information from the "Customers" table to display on the report. Select "Modify the Report's Design" on the last screen of the "Report Wizard" to change the layout of the report.

Step 5

Add a page header and footer, and include your company contact information, logo and invoice terms. Increase the size of the report's detail section to display only one transaction per page. Add subtotals and totals by placing calculated controls on your report and inputting an expression such as "=[BillableHours]*[Wage]."

Example

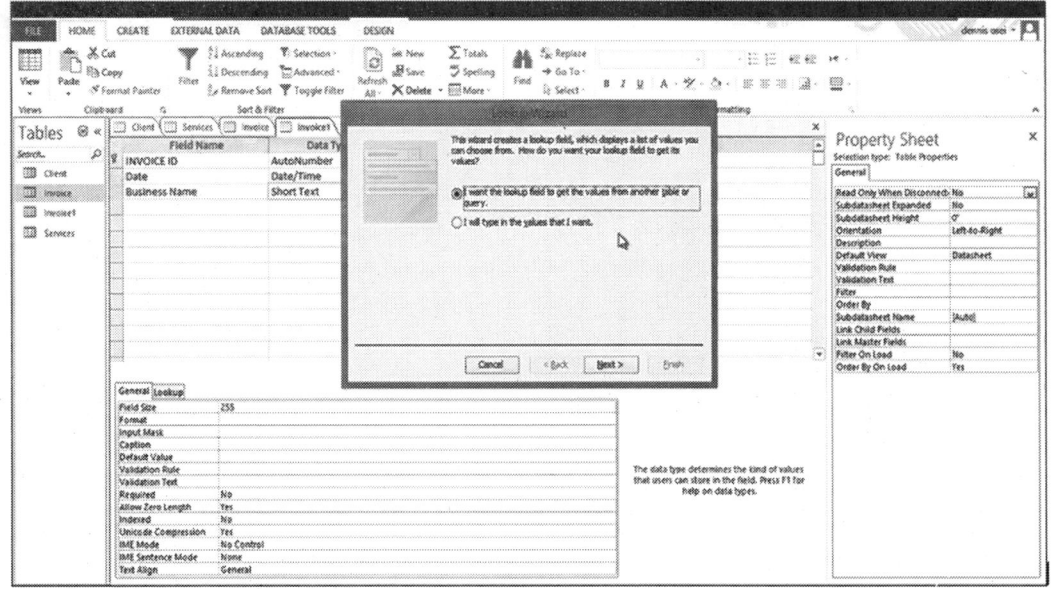

PRACTICAL 5

Drug information storage and retrieval using MS Access

INTRODUCTION

A database is an organized collection of data, generally stored and accessed electronically from a computer system. Where databases are more complex they are often developed using formal design and modeling techniques.

Database objects are the main players in an Access database. Altogether, we have six different types of database objects. From these we'll use Table to create database and Queries to retrieve the stored drug information.

Tables store information. Tables are the heart of any database, and you can create as many tables as you need to store different types of information. A drug databases of marketed drugs contain trade name, dosage form, and strength, they usually do not allocate a unit of prescription or route of administration to the trade name. Apart this, electronic dose calculation, the relation between the denominator of strength and prescribed unit also available software in coded form. When you want to review, add, change, or delete data from the database, consider using a query. Using a query, you can answer very specific questions about the data that would be difficult to answer by looking at table data directly. You can use queries to filter your data, to perform calculations with your data, and to summarize your data. You can also use queries to automate many data management tasks and to review changes in your data before you commit to those changes.

Creating a Table

Create a Table with by using the suitable fields and data type respectively. Visit page How to Create a database in MS Access to store the patient information with the required fields Using access to know more.

Creating Queries

1. On the Create tab, click Query Design.
2. In the Show Table dialog box, on the Tables tab, double.

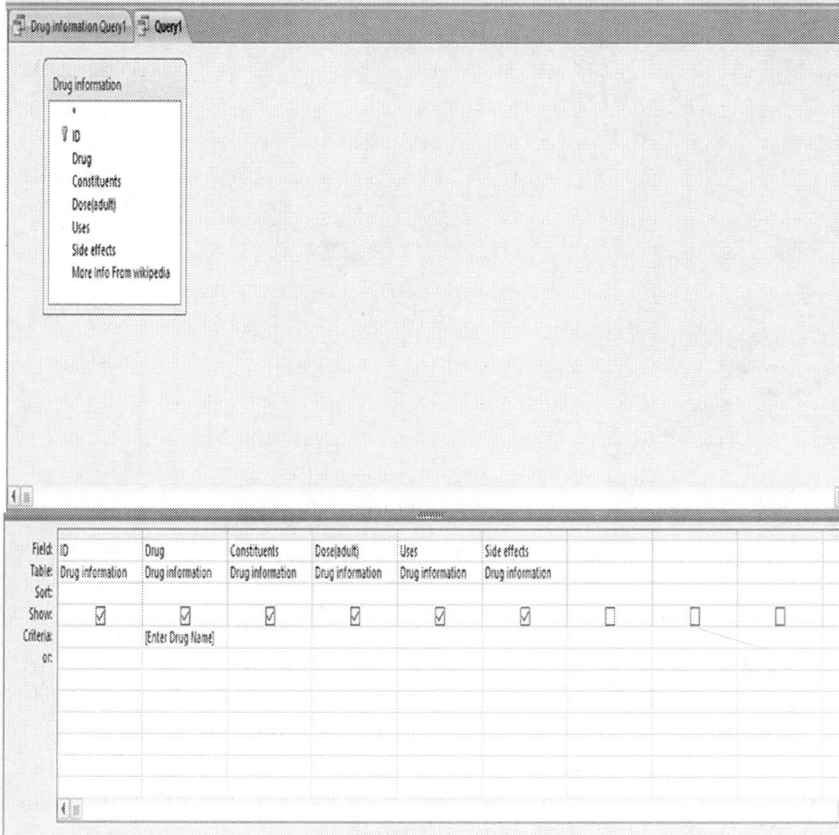

3. Click Products/Tables you created.

4. Close the Show Table dialog box.

5. In the Products table, double-click Fields to add these fields to the query design grid below (design grid: The grid that you use to design a query or filter in query Design view or in the Advanced Filter/Sort window. For queries, this grid was formerly known as the QBE grid.).

6. Add Criteria to field the you want to be asked on Query RUN, to show filtered record according to the query entered.

7. On the Design tab, in the Results group, click Run. Enter the Field Value and click OK.

The query runs, and then displays a list of Fields and their records. This is called retrieval of records.

PRACTICAL 6

Creating and working with queries in MS Access

The Query Design Button

Click the Query Design button to create a query in Design view. You could also use the Query Wizard button next to it to launch the Query Wizard; however, Design view gives you more control over the query.

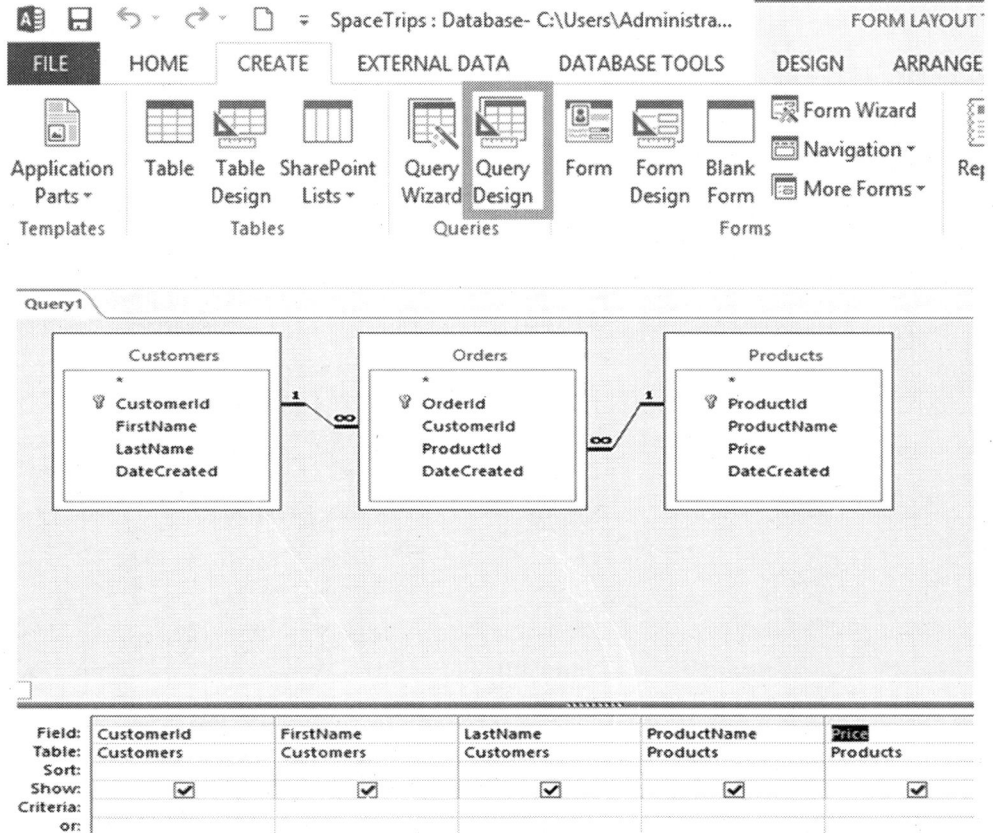

Query Design View

Query design view allows you to specify the precise criteria for the query. You can choose which tables are shown in the results, which fields to use, add filtering criteria, and more.

The Run Button

Clicking the Run button will run the query. Clicking the Datasheet view button next to it will also run the query.

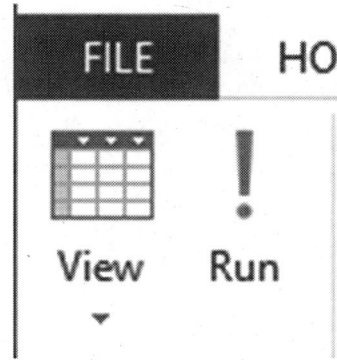

The Query Results

CustomerId	FirstName	LastName	ProductName	Price
1	Homer	Simpson	Venus Carrera ET	$190,000.99
2	Peter	Griffin	Mars Dreamliner 787	$82,000.00
10	Bender	Rodríguez	Mercury Riser 2020	$55,000.00
10	Bender	Rodríguez	Pluto Mini Racer	$25,000.00
3	Stewie	Griffin	Mars Daytripper	$35,000.00
4	Brian	Griffin	Venus Carrera ET	$190,000.99
5	Cosmo	Kramer	Mercury Riser 2020	$55,000.00
6	Philip	Fry	Saturn SUV	$65,750.00
7	Amy	Wong	Pluto Mini Racer	$25,000.00
8	Hubert J.	Farnsworth	Mars Dreamliner 787	$82,000.00
1	Homer	Simpson	Saturn SUV	$65,750.00
6	Philip	Fry	Venus Carrera ET	$190,000.99
* (New)				

Query1

The query results are displayed in Datasheet view.

Saving the Query

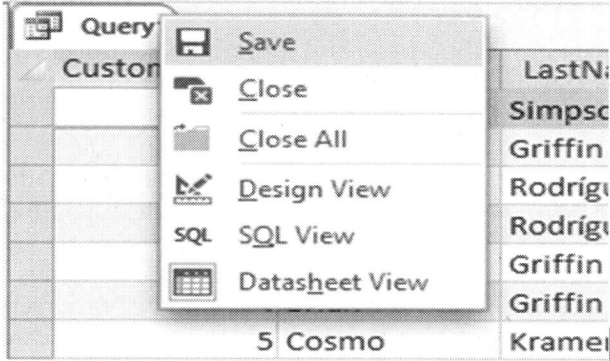

Saving a query.

Modifying the Query

You can go back and forth between Datasheet view and Design view to modify your query. Design view allows you to specify the exact criteria for your query.

For example, you might want the query to return only those products from a certain company. Or you might need a list of all users who have spent over a certain amount. The query Design view enables this and much more.

Field:	CustomerId	FirstName	LastName	ProductName	Price
Table:	Customers	Customers	Customers	Products	Products
Sort:					
Show:	✔	✔	✔	✔	✔
Criteria:					>80000
or:					

Design view allows you to add criteria with which to filter the results. Here, we've added criteria to filter the results to only those with a price over a certain amount (80000).

Result

CustomerId ▾	FirstName ▾	LastName ▾	ProductName ▾	Price ▾
1 Homer		Simpson	Venus Carrera ET	$190,000.99
2 Peter		Griffin	Mars Dreamliner 787	$82,000.00
4 Brian		Griffin	Venus Carrera ET	$190,000.99
8 Hubert J.		Farnsworth	Mars Dreamliner 787	$82,000.00
6 Philip		Fry	Venus Carrera ET	$190,000.99

Only records with a value greater than $80,000 are returned. This is because we specified >80000 in the Criteria field.

PRACTICAL 7

Exporting Tables, Queries, Forms and Reports to web pages

MS Access allows users to built a powerful integrated platforms of inserting, saving, retrieving the information into the database. There are many platforms for these facilities in MS Access, e.g. Tables, Queries, Forms, Reports, etc.

In previous posts we have learnt how to create the Tables, Queries, Forms and Reports, etc. But if we want to open the data into another application then it provides a way to do the same. We can export the table, queries, etc. into another format such as XML, web pages.

In this tutorial, you will come to know how to export the tables or queries into the web page format which allow you to open the table in web browsers.

If you don't know how to create the data tables, queries, and reports then please read those articles before it.

We just follow some easy steps to do the same as follow

Procedure:

1. Open a database table that is created previously or create a new database table.
2. Go to the External Data ribbon and click on More and then click on HTML Document in the Export group.
3. Now Click on browse to specify the destination of the file where you want to save it in your computer.
4. Select the Formatting option for the better look of the table and click OK.

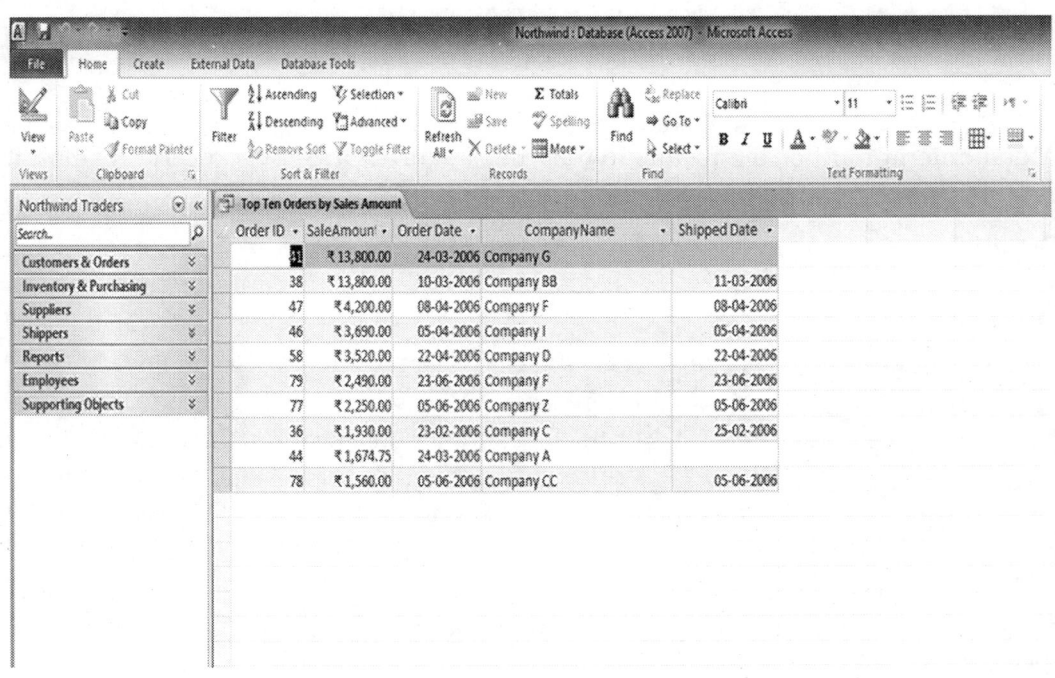

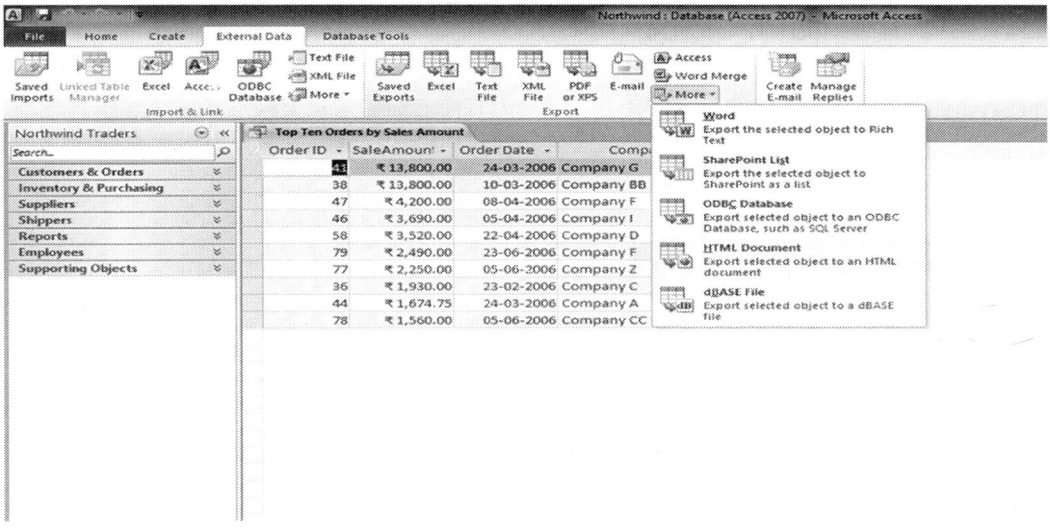

5. Now select the layout of the table, query form or report whatever you are exporting. For example, in case of table select either a HTML Template or choose encoding type of the HTML File. And click OK.

6. A popup window appear showing the message of finishing the exporting and option to save export steps. Simply click on Close.

7. Exporting Finished. Open the destination folder of the HTML file, and open the HTML File in the Web Browser.

8. Similarly follow step 1 to 5 to create HTML file for Queries, Forms and Report databases.

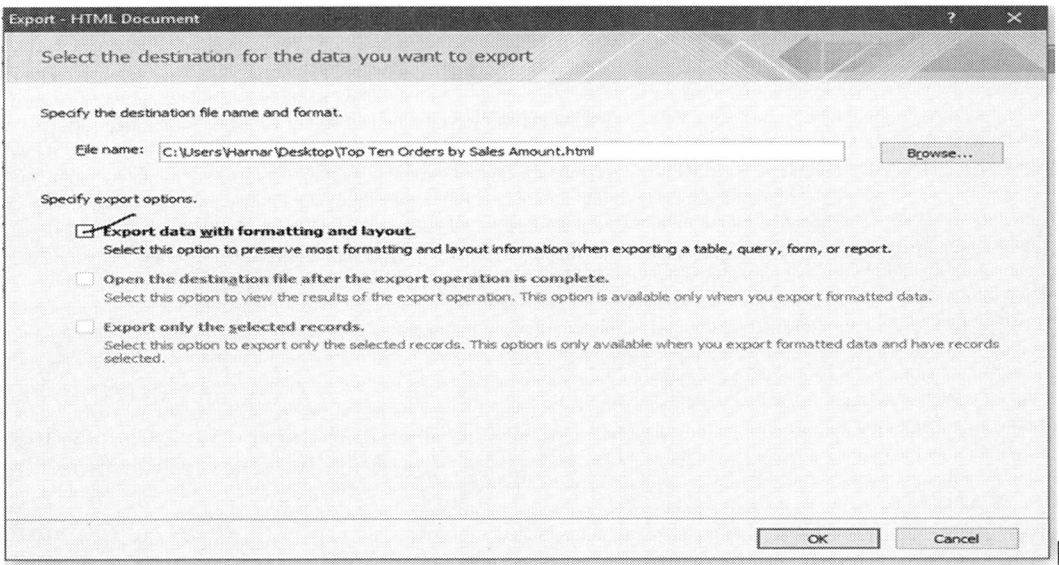

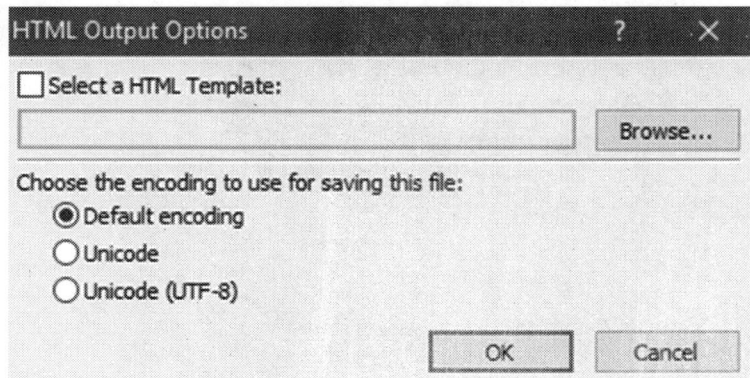

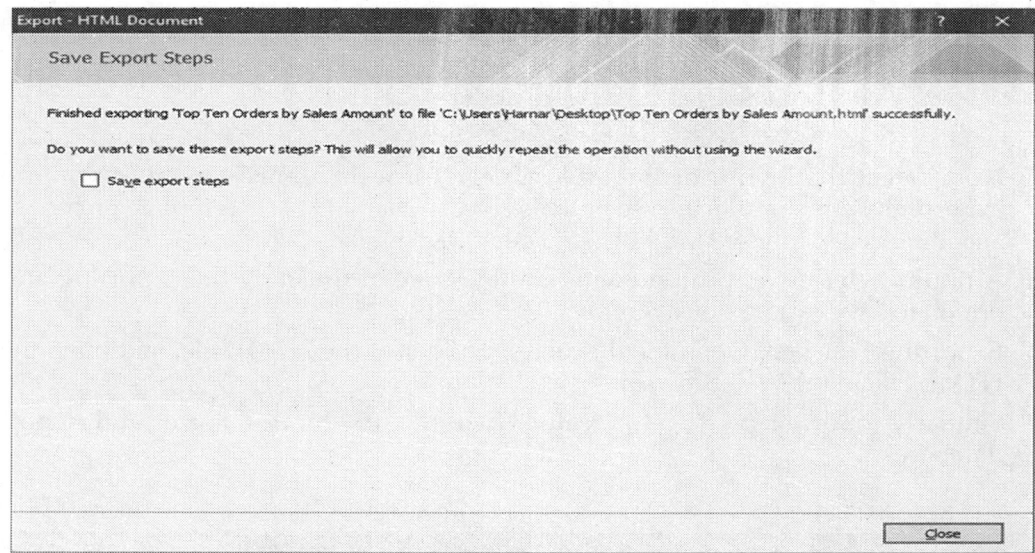

Exporting Tables, Queries, Forms and Reports to XML pages

XML and Access

Access exports several XML file types. The three XML export options produce the following XML file types:

1. Data (XML) produces an XML file.
2. Schema of the Data produces an XSD file.
3. Presentation of Your Data produces three files: an XML, an XSL, and an HTML file.

XML can share data, information on presenting that data, and schemas. In a relational database, schema refers to the tables. Specifically, schema identifies the fields and the relationships between fields and tables. Importing a schema can make creating a replica of a table much easier. In fact, you could quickly re-create the entire table structure using schema data.

You can export data or schema using the Access user interface or Visual Basic for Applications (VBA) code. To export schema manually:

1. Select a table in the Database window—for this example, we'll export the Customers (a table in Northwind, the sample database that comes with Access) schema.
2. Select Export from the File menu.
3. Name the XML file CustomersSchema.
4. Select XML as the file type in the Save As Type control. Don't type the XSD extension; XML will assign the right extension.
5. Click Export and Access will display three export options, as shown in Fig. 7.A: Data (XML), Schema Of The Data, and Presentation Of Your Data. The first two options are selected by default.
6. Choose Schema Of The Data; you're really just deselecting Data (XML).
7. Click the Advanced button. (You can omit details from the exported information, as shown in Fig. 7.B.) Don't make any changes right now, but you should know that you can omit primary key and index information from the exported file.
8. Click the Data tab and click OK.

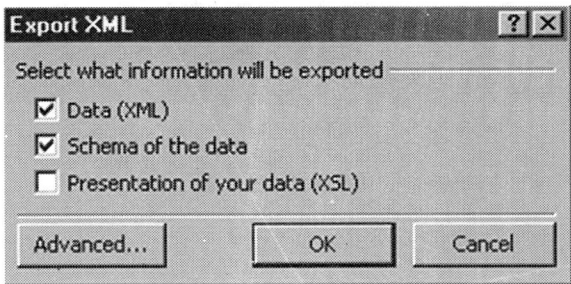

Fig. 7.A

Choose the schema of the data option to export schema to an XML file.

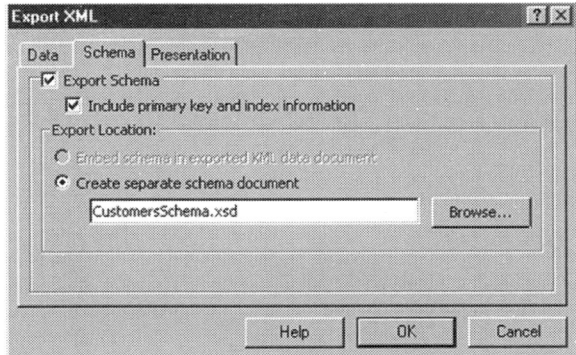

Fig. 7.B

The Advanced options let you omit details from the exported information.

You can learn a lot about an XSD schema file by viewing it in a browser. Figure 7.C shows CustomerSchema.xsd in Word. The file is really just text that contains details about the Customers table structure.

```xml
<?xml version="1.0" encoding="UTF-8"?>
<xsd:schema xmlns:xsd="http://www.w3.org/2000/10/XMLSchema"
xmlns:od="urn:schemas-microsoft-com:officedata">
<xsd:element name="dataroot">
<xsd:complexType>
<xsd:choice maxOccurs="unbounded">
<xsd:element ref="Customers"/>
</xsd:choice>
</xsd:complexType>
</xsd:element>
<xsd:element name="Customers">
<xsd:annotation>
<xsd:appinfo>
<od:index index-name="PrimaryKey" index-key="CustomerID " primary="yes"
unique="yes" clustered="no"/>
<od:index index-name="City" index-key="City " primary="no" unique="no"
clustered="no"/>
<od:index index-name="CompanyName" index-key="CompanyName " primary="no"
unique="no" clustered="no"/>
<od:index index-name="PostalCode" index-key="PostalCode " primary="no"
unique="no" clustered="no"/>
<od:index index-name="Region" index-key="Region " primary="no" unique="no"
clustered="no"/>
</xsd:appinfo>
</xsd:annotation>
```

Fig. 7.C

Open the XSD file in Word to see what it contains.

Glossary and Appendix

Application: Computer software that performs a task or set of tasks, such as word processing or drawing. Applications are also referred to as programs.

ASCII: American Standard Code for Information Interchange, an encoding system for converting keyboard characters and instructions into the binary number code that the computer understands.

Bandwidth: The capacity of a networked connection. Bandwidth determines how much data can be sent along the networked wires. Bandwidth is particularly important for Internet connections, since greater bandwidth also means faster downloads.

Binary code: The most basic language a computer understands, it is composed of a series of 0s and 1s. The computer interprets the code to form numbers, letters, punctuation marks, and symbols.

Bit: The smallest piece of computer information, either the number 0 or 1. In short they are called binary digits.

Browser: Software used to navigate the Internet. Google Chrome, Firefox, Netscape Navigator and Microsoft Internet Explorer are today's most popular browsers for accessing the World Wide Web.

Byte: Most computers use combinations of eight bits, called bytes, to represent one character of data or instructions. For example, the word **cat** has three characters, and it would be represented by three bytes.

Cache: A small data-memory storage area that a computer can use to instantly re-access data instead of re-reading the data from the original source, such as a hard drive. Browsers use a cache to store web pages so that the user may view them again without reconnecting to the Web.

Client: A single user of a network application that is operated from a server. A client/server architecture allows many people to use the same data simultaneously. The program's main component (the data) resides on a centralized server, with smaller components (user interface) on each client.

Cookie: A text file sent by a Web server that is stored on the hard drive of a computer and relays back to the Web server things about the user, his or her computer, and/or his or her computer activities.

CPU: Central Processing Unit. The brain of the computer.

Crash: A hardware or software problem that causes information to be lost or the computer to malfunction. Sometimes a crash can cause permanent damage to a computer.

Cursor: A moving position-indicator displayed on a computer monitor that shows a computer operator where the next action or operation will take place.

Database: A collection of similar information stored in a file, such as a database of addresses. This information may be created and stored in a database management system (DBMS).

Default: The pre-defined configuration of a system or an application. In most programs, the defaults can be changed to reflect personal preferences.

Desktop: The main directory of the user interface. Desktops usually contain icons that represent links to the hard drive, a network (if there is one), and a trash or recycling can for files to be deleted. It can also display icons of frequently used applications, as requested by the user.

Desktop publishing: The production of publication-quality documents using a personal computer in combination with text, graphics, and page layout programs.

Directory: A repository where all files are kept on computer.

Disk: *Two distinct types. The names refer to the media inside the container*:
A hard disc stores vast amounts of data. It is usually inside the computer but can be a separate peripheral on the outside. Hard discs are made-up of several rigid coated metal discs. Currently, hard discs can store 15 to 30 Gb (gigabytes).

A floppy disc, 3.5" square, usually inserted into the computer and can store about 1.4 megabytes of data. The 3.5" square floppies have a very thin, flexible disc inside. There is also an intermediate-sized floppy disc, trademarked Zip discs, which can store 250 megabytes of data.

Disk drive: The equipment that operates a hard or floppy disc.

Domain: Represents an IP (Internet Protocol) address or set of IP addresses that comprise a domain. The domain name appears in URLs to identify web pages or in email addresses. For example, the email address for the First Lady is first.lady@whitehouse.gov, whitehouse.gov, being the domain name. Each domain name ends with a suffix that indicates what top level domain it belongs to. These are : .com for commercial, .gov for government, .org for organization, .edu for educational institution, .biz for business, .info for information, .tv for television, .ws for website. Domain suffixes may also indicate the country in which the domain is registered. No two parties can ever hold the same domain name.

Domain name: The name of a network or computer linked to the Internet. Domains are defined by a common IP address or set of similar IP (Internet Protocol) addresses.

Download: The process of transferring information from a web site (or other remote location on a network) to the computer. It is possible to download a file which include text, image, audio, video and many others.

DOS: Disk Operating System. An operating system designed for early IBM-compatible PCs.

Drop-down menu: A menu window that opens vertically on-screen to display context-related options. Also called pop-up menu or pull-down menu.

DVD: Digital Video Disc. Similar to a CD-ROM, it stores and plays both audio and video.

E-book: An electronic (usually hand-held) reading device that allows a person to view digitally stored reading materials.

Email: Electronic mail; messages, including memos or letters, sent electronically between networked computers that may be across the office or around the world.

Ethernet: A type of network.

Ethernet card: A board inside a computer to which a network cable can be attached.

File: A set of data that is stored in the computer.

Firewall: A set of security programs that protect a computer from outside interference or access via the Internet.

Folder: A structure for containing electronic files. In some operating systems, it is called a directory.

Fonts: Sets of typefaces (or characters) that come in different styles and sizes.

Gigabyte (GB): 1024 megabytes. Also called gig.

Gopher: An Internet search tool that allows users to access textual information through a series of menus, or if using FTP, through downloads.

GUI: Graphical user interface, a system that simplifies selecting computer commands by enabling the user to point to symbols or illustrations (called icons) on the computer screen with a mouse.

Hard copy: A paper printout of what you have prepared on the computer.

Hard drive: Another name for the hard disc that stores information in a computer.

Hardware: The physical and mechanical components of a computer system, such as the electronic circuitry, chips, monitor, disks, disk drives, keyboard, modem, and printer.

Home page: The main page of a Web site used to greet visitors, provide information about the site, or to direct the viewer to other pages on the site.

HTML: Hypertext markup language, a standard of text markup conventions used for documents on the World Wide Web. Browsers interpret the codes to give the text structure and formatting (such as bold, blue, or italic).

HTTP: Hypertext transfer protocol, a common system used to request and send HTML documents on the World Wide Web. It is the first portion of all URL addresses on the World Wide Web.

HTTPS: Hypertext transfer protocol secure, often used in intracompany internet sites. Passwords are required to gain access.

Hyperlink: Text or an image that is connected by hypertext coding to a different location. By selecting the text or image with a mouse, the computer jumps to (or displays) the linked text.

Hypermedia: Integrates audio, graphics, and/or video through links embedded in the main program.

Hypertext: A system for organizing text through links, as opposed to a menu-driven hierarchy such as Gopher. Most Web pages include hypertext links to other pages at that site, or to other sites on the World Wide Web.

Icons: Symbols or illustrations appearing on the computer screen that indicate program files or other computer functions.

Input: Data that goes into a computer device.

Input device: A device, such as a keyboard, stylus and tablet, mouse, puck, or microphone, that allows input of information (letters, numbers, sound, video) to a computer.

Instant messaging (IM): A chat application that allows two or more people to communicate over the Internet via real-time keyed-in messages.

Interface: The interconnections that allow a device, a program, or a person to interact. Hardware interfaces are the cables that connect the device to its power source and to other devices. Software interfaces allow the program to communicate with other programs (such as the operating system), and user interfaces allow the user to communicate with the program (e.g. via mouse, menu commands, icons, voice commands, etc.).

Internet: An international conglomeration of interconnected computer networks. Begun in the late 1960s, it was developed in the 1970s to allow government and university researchers to share information. The Internet is not controlled by any single group or organization. Its original focus was research and communications, but it continues to expand, offering a wide array of resources for business and home users.

IP (Internet Protocol) address: An Internet Protocol address is a unique set of numbers used to locate another computer on a network. The format of an IP address is a 32-bit string of four numbers separated by periods. Each number can be from 0 to 255 (i.e. 1.154.10.255). Within a closed network IP addresses may be assigned at random, however, IP addresses of web servers must be registered to avoid duplicates.

Java: An object-oriented programming language designed specifically for programs (particularly multimedia) to be used over the Internet. Java allows programmers to create small programs or applications (applets) to enhance Web sites.

JavaScript/ECMA script: A programming language used almost exclusively to manipulate content on a web page. Common JavaScript functions include validating forms on a web page, creating dynamic page navigation menus, and image rollovers.

Kilobyte (K or KB): Equal to 1,024 bytes.

Linux: A UNIX-like, open-source operating system developed primarily by Linus Torvalds. Linux is free and runs on many platforms, including both PCs and Macintoshes. Linux is an open-source operating system, meaning that the source code of the operating system is freely available to the public. Programmers may redistribute and modify the code, as long as they don't collect royalties on their work or deny access to their code. Since development is not restricted to a single corporation more programmers can debug and improve the source code faster.

Laptop and notebook: Small, lightweight, portable battery-powered computers that can fit onto your lap. They each have a thin, flat, liquid crystal display screen.

Macro: A script that operates a series of commands to perform a function. It is set up to automate repetitive tasks.

Mac OS: An operating system with a graphical user interface, developed by Apple for Macintosh computers. Current System X.1.(10) combines the traditional Mac interface with a strong underlying UNIX. Operating system for increased performance and stability.

Megabyte (MB): Equal to 1,048,576 bytes, usually rounded off to one million bytes (also called a meg).

Memory: Temporary storage for information, including applications and documents. The information must be stored to a permanent device, such as a hard disc or CD-ROM before the power is turned off, or the information will be lost. Computer memory is measured in terms of the amount of information it can store, commonly in megabytes or gigabytes.

Menu: A context-related list of options that users can choose from.

Menu bar: The horizontal strip across the top of an application's window. Each word on the strip has a context sensitive drop-down menu containing features and actions that are available for the application in use.

Merge: To combine two or more files into a single file.

MHz: An abbreviation for **Megahertz,** or **one million hertz.** One MHz represents one million clock cycles per second and is the measure of a computer microprocessor's speed. For example, a microprocessor that runs at 300 MHz executes 300 million cycles per second. Each instruction a computer receives takes a fixed number of clock cycles to carry out, therefore the more cycles a computer can execute per second, the faster its programs run. Megahertz is also a unit of measure for bandwidth.

Microprocessor: A complete central processing unit (CPU) contained on a single silicon chip.

Minimize: A term used in a GUI operating system that uses windows. It refers to reducing a window to an icon, or a label at the bottom of the screen, allowing another window to be viewed.

Modem: A device that connects two computers together over a telephone or cable line by converting the computer's data into an audio signal. Modem is a contraction for the process it performs: modulate-demodulate.

Monitor: A video display terminal.

Mouse: A small hand-held device, similar to a trackball, used to control the position of the cursor on the video display; movements of the mouse on a desktop correspond to movements of the cursor on the screen.

MP3: Compact audio and video file format. The small size of the files makes them easy to download and e-mail. Format used in portable playback devices.

Multimedia: Software programs that combine text and graphics with sound, video, and animation. A multimedia PC contains the hardware to support these capabilities.

MS-DOS: An early operating system developed by Microsoft Corporation (Microsoft Disc Operating System).

Network: A system of interconnected computers.

Open source: Computer programs whose original source code was revealed to the general public so that it could be developed openly. Software licensed as open source can be freely changed or adapted to new uses, meaning that the source code of the operating system is freely available to the public. Programmers may redistribute and modify the code, as long as they don't collect royalties on their work or deny access to their code. Since development is not restricted to a single corporation more programmers can debug and improve the source code faster.

Operating system: A set of instructions that tell a computer on how to operate when it is turned on. It sets up a filing system to store files and tells the computer how to display information on a video display. Most PC operating systems are DOS (disc operated system) systems, meaning the instructions are stored on a disc (as opposed to being originally stored in the microprocessors of the computer). Other well-known operating systems include UNIX, Linux, Macintosh, and Windows.

Output: Data that come out of a computer device. For example, information displayed on the monitor, sound from the speakers, and information printed to paper.

Palm: A hand-held computer.

PC: Personal computer. Generally refers to computers running Windows with a Pentium processor.

PC board: Printed circuit board, a board printed or etched with a circuit and processors. Power supplies, information storage devices, or changers are attached.

PDA: Personal digital assistant, a hand-held computer that can store daily appointments, phone numbers, addresses, and other important information. Most PDAs link to a desktop or laptop computer to download or upload information.

PDF: Portable document format, a format presented by Adobe Acrobat that allows documents to be shared over a variety of operating systems. Documents can contain words and pictures and be formatted to have electronic links to other parts of the document or to places on the web.

Pentium chip: Intel's fifth generation of sophisticated high-speed microprocessors. Pentium means the fifth element.

Peripheral: Any external device attached to a computer to enhance operation. Examples include external hard drive, scanner, printer, speakers, keyboard, mouse, trackball, stylus and tablet, and joystick.

Personal computer (PC): A single-user computer containing a central processing unit (CPU) and one or more memory circuits.

Petabyte: A measure of memory or storage capacity and is approximately a thousand terabytes.

Platform: The operating system, such as UNIX, Macintosh, Windows, on which a computer is based.

Plug and play: Computer hardware or peripherals that come set up with necessary software so that when attached to a computer, they are recognized by the computer and are ready to use.

Pop-up menu: A menu window that opens vertically or horizontally on-screen to display context-related options. Also called drop-down menu or pull-down menu.

Power PC: A competitor of the Pentium chip. It is a new generation of powerful sophisticated microprocessors produced from an Apple-IBM-Motorola alliance.

Printer: A mechanical device for printing a computer's output on paper. There are three major types of printer:
- **Dot matrix**—creates individual letters, made up of a series of tiny ink dots, by punching a ribbon with the ends of tiny wires. (This type of printer is most often used in industrial settings, such as direct mail for labelling.)
- **Ink jet**—sprays tiny droplets of ink particles onto paper.
- **Laser**—uses a beam of light to reproduce the image of each page using a magnetic charge that attracts dry toner that is transferred to paper and sealed with heat.

Program: A precise series of instructions written in a computer language that tells the computer what to do and how to do it. Programs are also called software or applications.

Programming language: A series of instructions written by a programmer according to a given set of rules or conventions (syntax). High-level programming languages are independent of the device on which the application (or program) will eventually run; low-level languages are specific to each program or platform. Programming language instructions are converted into programs in language specific to a particular machine or operating system (machine language). So that the computer can interpret and carry-out the instructions. Some common programming languages are BASIC, C, C++, dBASE, FORTRAN, and Perl.

Push technology: Internet tool that delivers specific information directly to a user's desktop, eliminating the need to surf for it. PointCast, which delivers news in user-defined categories, is a popular example of this technology.

Quick time: Audiovisual software that allows movie-delivery via the Internet and e-mail. QuickTime images are viewed on a monitor.

RAID: Redundant array of inexpensive disks, a method of spreading information across several disks set-up to act as a unit, using two different techniques:

- **Disk striping**—storing a bit of information across several discs (instead of storing it all on one disc and hoping that the disc doesn't crash).
- **Disk mirroring**—simultaneously storing a copy of information on another disc so that the information can be recovered if the main disc crashes.

RAM: Random access memory, one of two basic types of memory. Portions of programs are stored in RAM when the program is launched so that the program will run faster. Though a PC has a fixed amount of RAM, only portions of it will be accessed by the computer at any given time. Also called memory.

Right-click: Using the right mouse button to open context-sensitive drop-down menus.

ROM: Read-only memory, one of two basic types of memory. ROM contains only permanent information put thereby the manufacturer. Information in ROM cannot be altered, nor can the memory be dynamically allocated by the computer or its operator.

Scanner: An electronic device that uses light-sensing equipment to scan paper images such as text, photos, and illustrations and translate the images into signals that the computer can then store, modify, or distribute.

Search engine: Software that makes it possible to look for and retrieve material on the Internet, particularly the Web. Some popular search engines are Alta Vista, Google, HotBot, Yahoo!, Web Crawler, and Lycos.

Server: A computer that shares its resources and information with other computers, called clients, on a network.

Software: Computer programs; also called applications.

Spider: A process search engines use to investigate new pages on a web site and collect the information that needs to be put in their indices.

Spreadsheet: Software that allows one to calculate numbers in a format that is similar to pages in a conventional ledger.

Storage: Devices used to store massive amounts of information so that it can be readily retrieved. Devices include RAIDs, CD-ROMs, DVDs.

Streaming: Taking packets of information (sound or visual) from the Internet and storing it in temporary files to allow it to play in continuous flow.

Surfing: Exploring the Internet.

Telnet: A way to communicate with a remote computer over a network.

Trackball: Input device that controls the position of the cursor on the screen; the unit is mounted near the keyboard, and movement is controlled by moving a ball.

Terabytes (TB): A thousand gigabytes.

UNIX: A very powerful operating system used as the basis of many high-end computer applications.

Upload: The process of transferring information from a computer to a web site (or other remote location on a network). To transfer information from a computer to a web site (or other remote location on a network).

URL: Uniform resource locator:
* The protocol for identifying a document on the Web.
* A Web address (e.g. www.tutorialspoint.com). A URL is unique to each user. See also domáin.

UPS: Uninterruptible power supply. An electrical power supply that includes a battery to provide enough power to a computer during an outage to back-up data and properly shut down.

USB: Universal serial bus. A multiple-socket USB connector that allows several USB-compatible devices to be connected to a computer.

USENET: A large unmoderated and unedited bulletin board on the Internet that offers thousands of forums, called newsgroups. These range from newsgroups exchanging information on scientific advances to celebrity fan clubs.

User friendly: A program or device whose use is intuitive to people with a non-technical background.

Video teleconferencing: A remote "face-to-face chat," when two or more people using a webcam and an Internet telephone connection chat online. The webcam enables both live voice and video.

Virtual reality (VR): A technology that allows one to experience and interact with images in a simulated three-dimensional environment. For example, you could design a room in a house on your computer and actually feel that you are walking around in it even though it was never built. (The Holodeck in the science-fiction TV series Star Trek : Voyager would be the ultimate virtual reality.) Current technology requires the user to wear a special helmet, viewing goggles, gloves, and other equipment that transmits and receives information from the computer.

Virus: An unauthorized piece of computer code attached to a computer program or portions of a computer system that secretly copies itself from one computer to another by shared discs and over telephone and cable lines. It can destroy information stored on the computer, and in extreme cases, can destroy operability. Computers can be protected from viruses if the operator utilizes good virus prevention software and keeps the virus definitions up to date. Most viruses are not programmed to spread themselves. They have to be sent to another computer by e-mail, sharing, or applications. The worm is an exception, because it is programmed to replicate itself by sending copies to other computers listed in the e-mail address book in the computer. There are many kinds of viruses, e.g.:
* Boot viruses place some of their code in the start-up disk sector to automatically execute when booting. Therefore, when an infected machine boots, the virus loads and runs.
* File viruses attached to program files (files with the extension.exe). When you run the infected program, the virus code executes.
* Macroviruses copy their macros to templates and/or other application document files.
* Trojan Horse is a malicious, security-breaking program that is disguised as something being such as a screen saver or game.
* Worm launches an application that destroys information on your hard drive. It also sends a copy of the virus to everyone in the computer's e-mail address book.

WAV: A sound format (pronounced wave) used to reproduce sounds on a computer.

Webcam: A video camera/computer set-up that takes live images and sends them to a Web browser.

Window: A portion of a computer display used in a graphical interface that enables users to select commands by pointing to illustrations or symbols with a mouse. "Windows" is also the name Microsoft adopted for its popular operating system.

World Wide Web ("WWW" or "the Web"): A network of servers on the Internet that use hypertext-linked databases and files. It was developed in 1989 by Tim Berners-Lee, a British computer scientist, and is now the primary platform of the Internet. The feature that distinguishes the Web from other Internet applications is its ability to display graphics in addition to text.

Word processor: A computer system or program for setting, editing, revising, correcting, storing, and printing text.

WYSIWYG: What You See Is What You Get. When using most word processors, page layout programs (See desktop publishing), and web page design programs, words and images will be displayed on the monitor as they will look on the printed page or web page.

Index